Praises

"This must-read book delivers case reports of amazing recoveries from neurological disorders for which conventional medicine has little to nothing to offer.

Neuro-Acupuncture applied by Dr. Jason Hao is nothing short of a miracle for patients. Many have complete resolution of complicated disease or injury. If you are a healthcare provider, learning this unique type of treatment will be a game changer in your practice. If you are a patient, this book will bring you hope for a life changing experience.

I have personally witnessed hundreds of patients recover using Dr. Hao's specialized technique."

—Sunil Pai MD

The Author of "An Inflammation Nation", *Founder & Medical Director, House of Sanjevani Integrative Medicine Healthy & Lifestyle Center, and VP of Neuro-Acupuncture Institute*

"This wonderful readable, accessible book introduces readers to the miracles of neuro-acupuncture, the new kid on the block as a treatment for neurological disorders.

I have personally met with patients Dr. Jason Hao had applied a few needles to. They shared their ability to regain partial or total mobility and speech when their case was explained to be incurable. In 120 pages Dr. Hao brings the light of hope and help to the darkness of affliction and hopelessness.

Recently, he has added "long covid" to the list of treatable disorders. At the Neuro-Acupuncture Institute, he continues to train practitioners who are dedicated to the goal of offering relief, understanding, and potential healing to a wider public and to western physicians."

—Judith Fein

Cultural Adventurer, Award-Winning International Travel Writer and Journalist, Speaker, and Author of "Life is a Trip: The Transformative Magic of Travel," "The Spoon from Minkowitz: A Bittersweet Roots Journey to Ancestral Lands" *to name a few.*

PRAISES

"Dr. Jason Hao's impactful book, *Hao Neuro-Acupuncture Restores Life,* is a comprehensive volume of genius. The master healer brilliantly shares his forty years of wisdom and expertise, as one of the world's foremost educators and providers of ancient Chinese acupuncture practices.

This book, the first of a series, is a vault of essential knowledge to guide readers with a deeper understanding to the incredible results and possibilities achieved by Dr. Hao, and most importantly, his patients.

Masterfully written and thoughtfully presented, it is an absolute must read for all who long to explore the life healing traditions and outcomes Dr. Hao has been inspired to share with the world. His patient results I have personally observed for many years, are so profound and so amazing, I do not have the words to accurately honor them. Possibly? .... "other worldly"."

—SCOTT CHRISTOPHER

International Awarded Artist, Professional Baseball Champion, and Author of "Baseball, Art, and Dreams"

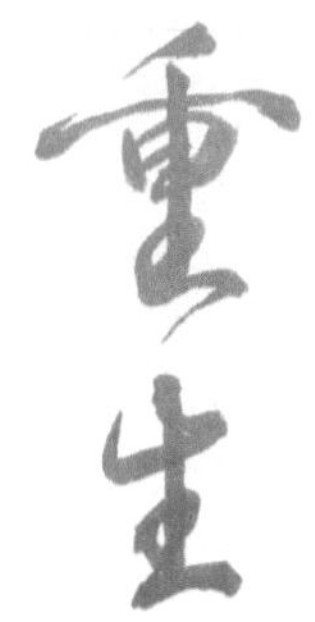

Hao Neuro-Acupuncture Restores *Life*

A New Treatment Is Born to Help Patients Suffering from Neurological Disorders

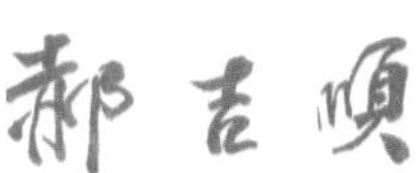

JASON JISHUN HAO, DOM

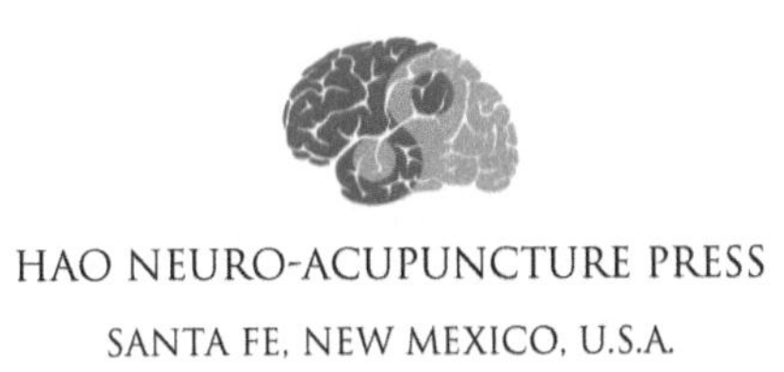

HAO NEURO-ACUPUNCTURE PRESS

SANTA FE, NEW MEXICO, U.S.A.

Hao Neuro-Acupuncture Restores Life
A New Treatment is Born to Help Patients
Suffering from Neurological Disorders
© 2023 by Jason Jishun Hao, DOM
Hao Neuro-Acupuncture Press, Santa Fe, NM
HaoNeuro-AcupuncturePress.com

PUBLISHER'S CATALOGING-IN-PUBLICATION

Names: Jishun Hao, Jason, author, illustrator.

Title: Hao neuro-acupuncture restores life : a new treatment is born to help patients suffering from neurological disorders / Jason Jishun Hao, DOM.

Description: Santa Fe, New Mexico, USA : Hao Neuro-Acupuncture Press, [2023] | Includes index.

Identifiers: ISBN: 979-8-9880219-0-2 (paperback) | 979-8-9880219-1-9 (hardback) | 979-8-9880219-2-6 (ebook) | LCCN: 2023917683

Subjects: LCSH: Acupuncture--Therapeutic use. | Nervous system--Diseases--Alternative treatment. | Brain--Diseases--Alternative treatment. | Neuromuscular diseases--Alternative treatment. | Pain--Alternative treatment. | Disabilities--Alternative treatment. | Alternative medicine. | Medicine, Chinese. | Paralysis--Alternative treatment--Case studies. | Aphasia--Alternative treatment--Case studies. | Cerebrovascular disease--Alternative treatment--Case studies. | Multiple sclerosis--Alternative treatment--Case studies. | Cerebral palsy--Alternative treatment--Case studies. | Autism--Alternative treatment--Case studies. | Brain--Wounds and injuries--Alternative treatment--Case studies. | Post COVID-19 condition (Disease)-- Alternative treatment--Case studies. | BISAC: MEDICAL / Acupuncture. | MEDICAL / Pain Management. | HEALTH & FITNESS / Diseases & Conditions / Nervous System (incl. Brain) | EDUCATION / Schools / Levels / Higher.

Classification: LCC: RM184 J57 2023 | DDC: 615.8/92--dc23

Artwork and Calligraphy: Jason Jishun Hao, DOM
Editing: Jeff Braucher
Cover and Book Design: Diane Rigoli
Printed in the United States of America

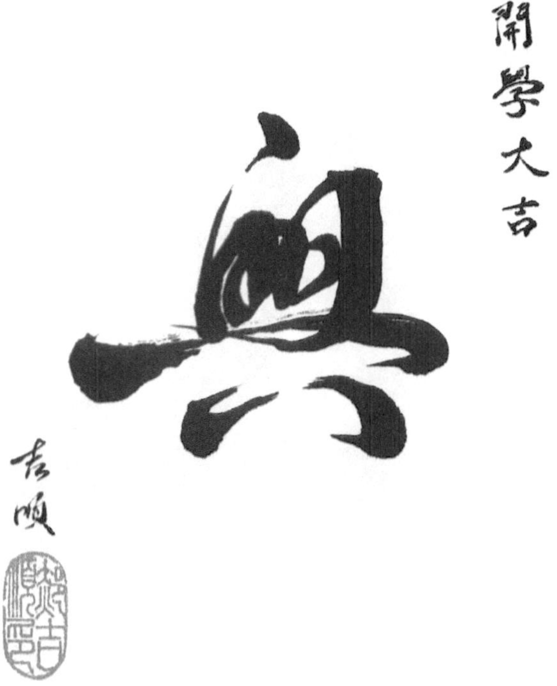

This book is dedicated to my parents
and all my teachers.

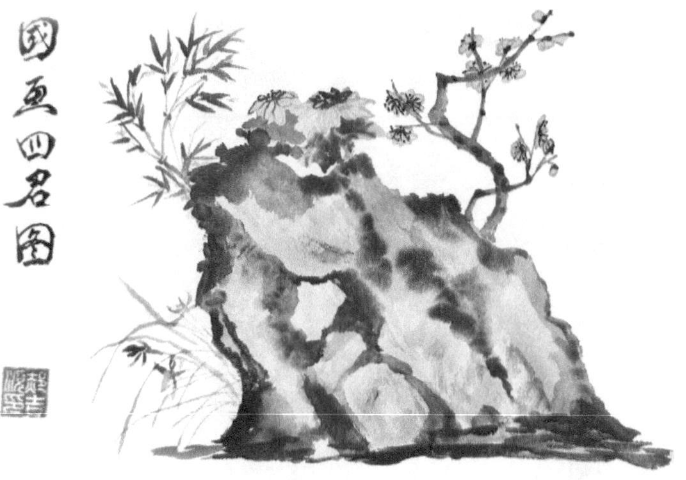

Because of their beauty, the plum flower, orchid, bamboo, and chrysanthemum have been common subjects in traditional Chinese ink and wash painting since the time of the Song dynasty (AD 960–1279) and later became popular with artists in Korea, Japan, and Vietnam. Each symbolizes one of the four seasons—the plum flower for winter, the orchid for spring, the bamboo for summer, and the chrysanthemum for autumn—and represents characteristics to aspire to.

CONTENTS

"A good doctor has the wings of angels hidden in his heart, and he opens his wings to care for every patient with the wings of love."

—Jason Jishun Hao, DOM

Foreword

I am a medical doctor who met Jason Hao DOM when I moved to Santa Fe, NM. After finishing medical school and a residency in Internal Medicine in the 1980s I met Dr. Hao while teaching western physiology at Southwest Acupuncture College (SWAC) in Santa Fe and became a patient of Drs. Jason and Linda Hao. In 2005 I had a serious bicycling accident associated with 10 cracked ribs, a collar-bone broken in 5 places, and temporary amnesia. Dr. Hao treated me with neuro-acupuncture 1 -2 times a week for more than three months and provided an invaluable support in my recovery.

This book: *Hao Neuro-Acupuncture Restores Life* offers readers insight into how neuro-acupuncture can help patients with neurological disorders. Neuro-acupuncture (also known as Scalp Acupuncture) has been a branch of traditional Chinese Acupuncture (TCM) and traditional East Asian Medicine (EAM) since the 1950s, explicitly integrating neurological diagnostic criteria with acupuncture therapeutics. It has shown promising short and long-term therapeutic outcomes. The neurological conditions for which neuro-acupuncture is used and about which published scientific information in available include: cerebral palsy, complex regional pain syndrome, chronic pain, stroke, multiple sclerosis (MS), autism spectrum disorders, and covid; to name a few of the commonly treated conditions with a neurological basis. Some of this scientific information is indexed in the National Library of Medicine database (NLM) and a search of the NLM databases using the terms "neuro-acupuncture" or "scalp acupuncture" yields almost five hundred citations.

Dr. Jason Jishun Hao DOM, MBA; earned his doctorate in Chinese Medicine in China between 1982 and 1987. Since his arrival in the United States in 1989 has been practicing, teaching, and involved in research and medical publishing. Dr. Hao is one of world's leading healthcare experts in Neuro-Acupuncture and in 2011 he co-authored with Dr. Linda Hao, a textbook on Chinese Scalp Acupuncture. He is one of the founders of the Neuro-Acupuncture Institute (NAI) in New Mexico and led the development of a multi-year, three-level training program for licensed acupuncture practitioners in neuro-acupuncture. This training covers both the theoretical and scientific basis for neuro-acupuncture as well as overseeing the delivery of neuro-acupuncture treatments that "restore life" to patients. He has trained hundreds of acupuncture practitioners and treated thousands of patients with disorders of the central nervous system around the world. In addition, Dr. Hao has taught neuro-acupuncture seminars at workshops sponsored by UCLA and Stanford University for more than a dozen years. In 2006 Dr. Hao successfully demonstrated neuro-acupuncture in treating a veteran suffering from phantom limb pain at Walter Reed Hospital in Washington DC.

Dr Hao has previously served as chairman of the National Certification Commission of Acupuncture and Oriental Medicine (NCCAOM) acupuncture committee and was the president of the board of directors at Southwest Acupuncture College (SWAC).

—DAVID RILEY, MD

Introduction

Chinese acupuncture has become increasingly popular during the past 50 years, particularly in the West, owing in part to its effectiveness in pain relief. Because of the growing number of scientific studies and clinical trials attesting to acupuncture's efficacy, in 1997 the National Institutes of Health (NIH) recommended teaching courses on it in medical schools. In fact, it is increasingly used as a viable treatment at university medical centers, usually in departments of anesthesia and pain management, including those at Harvard University, Stanford University, Johns Hopkins University, and University of California, Los Angeles. NIH also affirmed acupuncture's ability to relieve pain and nausea induced by surgery, chemotherapy, and morning sickness, and to treat and rehabilitate conditions such as headaches, strokes, and fibromyalgia. A more recent report published by the World Health Organization cited 31 maladies whose conditions had been improved by acupuncture in clinical trials.

Most of the 50 states in the US have laws regulating the practice of acupuncture, and coverage in health insurance policies is now commonly available. Research continues to identify new treatment options, which become the basis for updated insurance and reimbursement policies.

Though Western medicine initially offered acupuncture as a treatment for pain, it has been used in China to both prevent and treat a wide range of conditions and illnesses for approximately 3,000 years. Around 100 BCE it was codified into a system of diagnosis and treatment in *The Yellow Emperor's Classic of Internal Medicine.* It documents the channels through which the vital energy or life force (Qi) flows—knowledge passed down from practitioners of various traditions to their students over the course of centuries. In time, the practice of acupuncture became more specified, as in the needle insertion points, for instance. Eventually it took its place as standard practice in China, along with herbs, massage, diet, and exercise.

In recent decades, acupuncture has evolved even further by adopting modern technology and science into its practice and developing additional methods of treatment, such as electric and laser acupuncture and new insertion points. This book describes the most profound development in Chinese acupuncture in the past 50 years: integrating modern Western medical knowledge of neuroanatomy, neurology, neuroscience, and neurological rehabilitation with ancient Chinese needling methods and scalp acupuncture to create a new technique called neuro-acupuncture.

Clinical studies have shown that neuro-acupuncture is the most effective practice for treating neurological disorders such as stroke, multiple sclerosis, Parkinson's disease, traumatic brain injury, phantom pain, cerebral palsy, autism, and even long COVID-19 symptoms. With the insertion of just a few needles, neuro-acupuncture can bring about extraordinary results—often immediate improvements and sometimes in a matter of several minutes.

Neuro-acupuncture treatments include needling in the scalp and ears, as well as the more common body acupuncture. Because it's a relatively new tool and not widely known for treating neurological disorders, it's difficult for Western medical practitioners and the general public to believe that an alternative method exists that can aid tremendously in recovery from disorders that have been so difficult if not impossible to treat in the past.

I have been practicing, researching, and teaching neuro-acupuncture and Chinese medicine for 40 years. Since 1989, in the US and Europe, I have taught neuro-acupuncture to practitioners of both Chinese and Western medicine who treat patients using acupuncture. This book includes several case studies from my clinical practice and seminars spanning the past four decades. For example, I applied neuro-acupuncture to treat seven veterans with excruciating phantom limb pain in 2006 at Walter Reed National Military Medical Center near Washington, DC.[1] In some cases, the pain was so intense and constant, they found it impossible to sleep. Each patient received only a single treatment. Three of them instantly felt complete relief from the pain, three others reported having very little pain after treatment, and only one patient showed no improvement. Such extraordinary results attest to the healing power of Neuro-Acupuncture.

This book is the first in a series intended to give information about neuro-acupuncture to a wider audience, both for the general public—especially those who are suffering from the disorders covered here—and those in medical professions. Some common central nervous system disorders are discussed in detail, showing how the treatments delivered highly effective results.

Each of the twelve case histories included in this book reflect my own clinical experience, as well as my thought processes, strategies, and special techniques in treating patients suffering from disorders of the central nervous system. Whenever possible, other modalities complementary to the neuro-acupuncture therapies are discussed in the case studies. I hope I have succeeded in introducing and explaining the treatments such that anyone without a medical background can understand them.

I have presented some seemingly miraculous cases, such as a quadriplegic woman who, after only two Chinese scalp acupuncture sessions, completely recovered. Another woman was cured of aphasia after three treatments. These new techniques are exceptional, and it thrills me every time my application of them succeeds in relieving a patient of a horrible condition. But it's important to emphasize that due to a variety of factors, neuro-acupuncture isn't always an effective treatment for every patient, and positive results can vary in degree.

Before I came to the United States, I was among a group of students who studied these techniques under the direct instruction of three famous Chinese specialists: Jiao Shunfa, the brilliant founder of Jiao' scalp acupuncture; Sun Shentian, a grand master of acupuncture in China and an exceptional professor of scalp acupuncture research, and Yu Zhishun, a professor of scalp acupuncture development. And in the decades since then, I have garnered extensive and valuable experience.

My hope is that this book will serve as a guided tour into the vital new field of neuro-acupuncture, offering information and encouragement to patients seeking help in overcoming illness and pain. Students, practitioners, and teachers of acupuncture may be inspired to seek out further knowledge and experience to incorporate neuro-acupuncture into their current practice. Finally, I hope this book will serve as a stepping-stone toward a deeper understanding of the continuing need for research and development in the field of Chinese neuro-acupuncture.

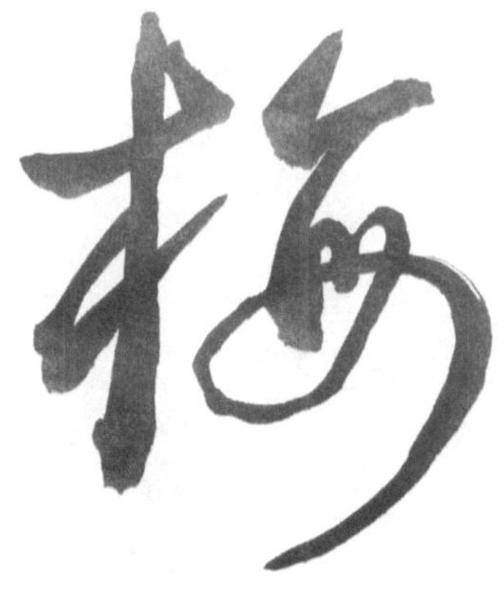

PART ONE

PLUM FLOWER

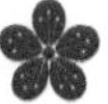

"Know yourself and your gifts, pursue excellence,
and serve others wholeheartedly."

—JASON JISHUN HAO, DOM

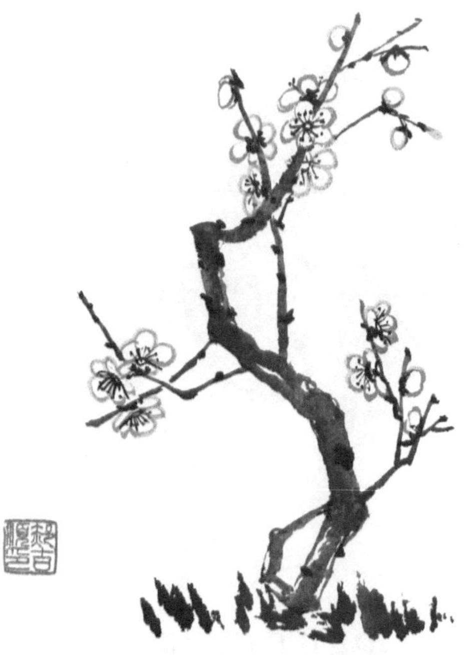

In the depth of winter, the plum tree blossoms despite the bitter cold. Thus, plum flowers depict resilience and perseverance, as well as inner beauty and humility. People paint plum flowers to bolster their courage when facing the harsh winter months and other types of adversity.

My Story: Coming to America

On September 23, 1989, my United Airlines flight was delayed eight hours because of heavy fog at the Shanghai airport. To me, the fog was like a blank canvas waiting for an artist to create a painting, and also like the future ahead of me—so much uncertainty and doubt. Finally, the plane lifted off the tarmac and I fell into a deep sleep, no longer able to remain awake.

With the sensory fog rolling in my mind, like a dream I felt as if I were walking on a cloud, flying as high as the plane, witnessing the bright and warm sunlight rising as we approached our destination. I was not able to get any REM sleep through the entire 18-hour flight from Shanghai to Los Angeles. There were too many interruptions and stops without any real food or drink. It was a very long flight.

That morning, 34 years ago, I was standing alone in the Los Angeles terminal, wearing an old brown polyester jacket, with a wrinkled photo of my lovely wife and three-year-old son and $80 in my pocket. I had mixed emotions: excited, sad, worried, anxious. I was in a new country that I wasn't sure would embrace what I had to offer.

In the parking lot of the airport, I noticed many handicap signs. I asked myself: Why are there so many disabled people? Isn't there any effective treatment for them? To me, each handicap sign represented a human being I could help. I felt compassion for those disabled people and a passionate desire to help them. I got excited and carried with me the hope for the patients who may not realize what is possible with brain plasticity and acupuncture.

Just a century ago scientists believed that any damage to the brain was permanent and untreatable. In the past 30 years we have learned that the brain has plasticity, meaning that a portion of the cerebral cortex can remap itself so some impaired neurological functions, even some damaged structures of the brain, can be restored by the right stimulation. Surgical methods can be invasive, but there is a way to tap into neuroplasticity without surgery, and that way is neuro-acupuncture.

Neuro-acupuncture is mostly unknown in the United States and in the West. For some people it is difficult to accept the reality that with just a few acupuncture needles and such a simple procedure, recovery from paralysis can occur. Neuro-acupuncture remaps the brain and makes it possible for the seated to stand, the silent to speak, and the paralyzed to walk.

In the past 40 years I have practiced neuro-acupuncture in China, the United States, and Europe. I have treated hundreds of people paralyzed in different areas of the body and have achieved excellent results. I have helped those patients get rid of their wheelchairs, walkers, crutches, and canes. The best results are astounding: A completely paralyzed two-year-old with cerebral palsy recovered with three neuro-acupuncture treatments. A 26-year-old quadriplegic woman recovered with only two treatments. An 80-year-old woman, whose stroke had caused aphasia and complete paralysis of her left side, fully recovered after 16 treatments.

Many newspapers, journals, and radio and television stations have reported the success of my treatments. These sources include the *Albuquerque Journal, Santa Fe New Mexican,* Walter Reed Medical Center's *Stripe, China Daily, Global Advances in Health and Medicine,* Fox News 14 in El Paso, and Global Dragon TV in Washington, DC.

Chapter One

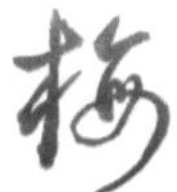

PARALYSIS

"Each handicap sign represents a
human being I could help."

—Jason Jishun Hao, DOM

PARALYSIS:
THE CONDITION AND DEFINITION

Paralysis is the partial or complete loss of voluntary movement and strength of one or more muscles. It may include the entire body, be limited to certain parts of the body, or follow a particular pattern. It is usually the result of injury or some other form of damage to the nervous system, especially the brain and spinal cord. If there is damage to the sensory nerves too, a loss of feeling can occur in the affected region along with the paralysis.

Aside from injury, major causes of paralysis include stroke, meningitis, encephalitis, poliomyelitis, amyotrophic lateral sclerosis (ALS), botulism, spinal bifida, and multiple sclerosis. The most common causes of paralysis I've seen in my acupuncture practice are stroke, multiple sclerosis, and traumatic injury of the brain or spinal cord. Cases resulting from damage of the nervous system are constant in their symptoms.

THE DIAGNOSIS

Classified by the affected areas of the body, the five types of paralysis are monoplegia, diplegia, hemiplegia, paraplegia, and quadriplegia. Monoplegia is impairment of only one limb. Diplegia affects the same area on both sides of the body, as in both arms or both legs. Hemiplegia impairs only one side of the body, as in the left arm, the left leg, and sometimes the left side of the facial muscles. Paraplegia is paralysis of both legs and the torso, and quadriplegia, also referred to as tetraplegia, is the partial or total loss of motor function of all limbs and the torso—the entire body below the neck.

Quadriplegia is often caused by severe brain damage, injury to the spinal cord, meningitis, polyneuritis, myasthenia gravis, progressive myodystrophy, multiple myositis, or acute infective multiple radiculoneuritis. In the case of spinal cord injury, the severity depends on both the degree of injury and the number of injured areas along the spinal cord. Whatever the cause, it can affect not only the limbs but the functioning of the torso, resulting in the loss or impairment in bowel and bladder control, sexual function, breathing, digestion, and other functions performed by the autonomic nervous system.

Quadriplegics may experience numbness, diminished sensation, or burning sensation and pain. Because of immobility and reduced functioning, they are susceptible to pressure sores, osteoporosis and fractures, blood clots, frozen joints, poor reflexes, spasticity, respiratory infections and other complications, and cardiovascular disease.

*"Yes, Doctor, it's me. I'm not paralyzed anymore,
and I walked here by myself."*

THE STORY

THE PATIENT

Barbara was brought in a wheelchair to a neuro-acupuncture seminar I conducted several years ago. She harbored little faith that any treatment could improve, let alone cure, her paralytic condition. Her quadriplegia was caused by a West Nile virus infection, and with loss of control of her body below the neck, she also had bowel and bladder incontinence.

Prior to her attendance at the seminar, she had tried many different healing modalities, none of which brought any improvement. She was understandably depressed. When I examined her, I found that all four limbs were tight and had spasms at times. Checking the muscular tone of her right arm, I determined that it ranked a grade of 2 out of a normal 6. Her left arm and both legs were completely paralyzed—a grade of 0 out of 6. Her tongue was red with a thin white coating; her pulse thready and wiry, which indicated to me that she had high stress due to her current condition. Her energy and blood flow was stagnated, with weakness in her limbs and internal organs.

THE CHALLENGE

While acupuncture on the body has been used to treat paralysis in China for centuries, the application of neuro-acupuncture as the foremost modality for this purpose is a relatively new concept. Lack of knowledge of its effectiveness causes Western doctors to assume it's a coincidence if a patient recovers from paralysis after acupuncture treatments.

It is imperative that doctors of Western medicine be made aware of the efficacy of neuro-acupuncture in the recovery from paralysis and other conditions. To accomplish this, it must be studied and perfected using modern science and technology. With a greater volume of clinical research, its potential can be fully explored and implemented effectively such that more and more doctors can become convinced of its efficacy, resulting in more paralyzed patients being able to reclaim their normal life and work.

THE RECOVERY

Barbara had extraordinary responses to her first neuro-acupuncture treatment. As soon as I inserted two needles in her scalp at specific points, the tightness in all four limbs loosened and the spasms disappeared. Soon after, she was able to move both arms and lift them. The Western physicians attending the seminar were astonished.

When I told Barbara that some similar patients were able to walk again, her eyes filled with tears.

I asked her, "What is your hope?"

"I want to be able to move my limbs and walk again."

After inserting four more needles into her scalp, I said, "You should be able to stand up," and encouraged her to try. She was amazed to find she had regained the ability to control her legs. Assisted by two people, nervously she stood up. When I urged her to start walking, she couldn't believe I was suggesting this.

With much excitement she followed my instruction and took one step, two steps, then three steps, and finally four steps. The audience applauded her courageous action.

Barbara held my hand for a long time, tears dripping down her face. She said, "Thank you so much, Doctor. You have given me hope to survive."

She received the same neuro-acupuncture treatment the next day and walked as much as she could, turning around about every 30 steps. She walked with confidence, a broad smile lighting her face.

During this second day, Barbara's fiancé spoke to me privately, asking, "What is the chance she'll recover completely?"

"She has a good chance of recovery, and that will more likely happen if she can continue getting acupuncture treatments and follow an intense exercise routine."

At another seminar in the same city months later, the physicians from the first seminar returned and eagerly waited to see how Barbara had progressed. When she walked into the conference room by herself, even I was astounded. I asked her, "Is that you, Barbara?"

"Yes, Doctor, it's me. I'm not paralyzed anymore, and I walked here by myself. Not only that, I got married and am back to work." We gave each other a hug and the audience applauded.

"How many treatments have you received since our sessions the last time I was here?"

"I haven't had any. My insurance wouldn't cover any more treatments, so I just followed the exercise routine you recommended." She ended with words I've heard from so many people: "It's like a miracle."

At the request of all of us attending the seminar, Barbara demonstrated with ease many kinds of movements of her four extremities, such as jumping, running, and raising her arms. All those actions prompted more enthusiastic applause from the audience.

I asked Barbara why she had returned to the second seminar. She said her only problem now was urgent, frequent urination and incontinence. Sometimes she had to use the restroom every twenty minutes. She added that she constantly felt pressure in her head and a "strange feeling" in her bladder. Hearing these details, I proceeded to put two needles on the top of her head (foot motor and sensory area) and two needles on the corners of her forehead (reproduction area). After this, only her third neuro-acupuncture treatment, Barbara left the seminar grateful and happy, no longer having that urgent feeling in her bladder, and able to hold her urine for up to two hours.

THE DISCUSSION

Neuro-acupuncture is frequently used in the recovery from paralysis due to stroke, multiple sclerosis, spinal cord injury, and traumatic brain injury. Proven to be effective in treating the types of paralysis already mentioned, it often brings about improvements quickly, sometimes in only one or two sessions for an astonishing degree of recovery. The hundreds of paralyzed patients in the US, China, and Europe whom I have helped are a testament to the remarkable results that can be achieved through neuro-acupuncture.

Treating quadriplegia is challenging. I need to emphasize how unusual it is that Barbara recovered completely after receiving only three treatments. It usually requires several months and sometimes even up to one to two years for patients to recover. And still only 70% of patients will improve.

Quadriplegia can be treated no matter how long a patient has endured the condition, but those who have been paralyzed fewer than three months show the greatest improvement. As a rule of thumb, the longer the period of impairment, the more gradual the improvement will be. For those with long-term quadriplegia, we need to be realistic about timing, but occasionally some patients will surprise practitioners by their speedy recovery.

Though many acupuncture points have been used to treat paralysis, scalp acupuncture offers the best and fastest response. Better recovery, however, requires other acupuncture techniques. For example, treatment in the limbs and torso has been shown to promote greater movement in the hands, fingers, feet, and toes.

If the practitioner is unable to rotate (twirl) the needle more than the required 200 times per minute, electrical stimulation serves as a viable option. Only two needles should be stimulated at any given scalp acupuncture session; otherwise, it confuses the brain to the point it can't respond. For body acupuncture, no more than two needles should be electrically stimulated in each limb. The best results tend to be reached by applying low frequency (for example, three hertz) with high intensity (when muscle contraction is visible). Another effective technique besides scalp acupuncture for treating quadriplegia is electrical stimulation applied above and below the damaged spinal area at *Huatuojiaji* points on the back along the spine.

Q&A

What are some of the main paralysis-causing disorders that neuro-acupuncture would work for?

In my practice I often see a paralyzed patient with one of the following disorders: stroke, traumatic brain injury, traumatic spinal injury, cerebral palsy, multiple sclerosis, Parkinson's disease, encephalitis, meningitis, poliomyelitis, acute myelitis, multiple neuritis, periodic paralysis, and ALS.

How frequently does a paralyzed patient need treatment?

I typically treat local patients 2–3 times per week for the first few weeks, then change treatments to 1–2 times per week. For patients coming from other states or countries, I usually treat them 4–5 times per week for 1–3 weeks, which will save them time as well as food and lodging expenses.

NOTES

*"Wheelchairs, crutches, and canes are
on sale at this acupuncture clinic."*

THE STORY

THE PATIENT

Julia was 49 years old when she was wheeled by a friend into our clinic in Santa Fe, New Mexico. Four months earlier, she was in a car accident, and her neck was severely damaged at the C-5 and C-6 spinal levels. When I examined her, I discovered she was paralyzed in all four limbs. She had minimal contraction and movement of her arm muscles, indicating that the muscular tone was a grade 2 out of a normal 6. Her hands, legs, and feet had a muscular tone of zero—complete paralysis. Julia also suffered urinary incontinence and experienced muscle spasms throughout her body. Her tongue was purplish with a thin, yellow, sticky coating. Her pulse showed weakness in the *Cun* and *Guan* positions, with faint pulses in the *Chi* position.

THE CHALLENGE

It's essential for paralyzed people to get acupuncture treatment as soon as possible in order to recover fully. Unfortunately, most of them are unaware of the beneficial results to be had through neuro-acupuncture. And many acupuncture practitioners have inadequate experience with the essential treatments. It is more difficult to achieve results for longtime paralyzed patients due to the likelihood of muscular atrophy and locked-up joints. For those with muscular atrophy, the sessions usually need to continue a long time, and sometimes acupuncture is not effective in helping them recover.

The Recovery

During her first treatment, as I was rapidly rotating the needles on her head, Julia felt instant relief from the muscle spasms. She told me that a sensation like electricity shot down her spine and radiated to her feet. As I applied more needle stimulation, she said, "I'm starting to feel a hot sensation in my hands and feet." She was so excited over these improvements, she started to cry.

"Can you wiggle your toes?" I asked.

"I'll try... Yes, look!"

"Wonderful! Your responses are an excellent prognosis that you will probably be able to stand up and walk during the third treatment." She was beaming.

In the third session, Julia was able to stand with the help of someone holding her knees, but she wasn't quite ready to walk. She also could lift her arms much higher. She told me her urinary incontinence had improved somewhat. From the third to the fifth visit, her limbs showed gradual improvements.

During the sixth treatment, she was able to kick her legs forcefully and also bend her legs and hold that position for a few minutes. I knew she should be able to stand and walk. "You can show major improvements today," I said, enthusiastically encouraging her as she struggled to get up on her feet and then stood with no support for one minute, two minutes, and then three minutes. This was just the beginning of exciting and dramatic results.

Following a rest, she stood up again and started taking some steps. It was a struggle, but Julia succeeded in walking 20 steps before she had to sit down, exhausted but excited. She told me some more good news: She had better control of her bladder and was able to hold her urine for six hours during the night.

After her eighth treatment, her body spasms were almost entirely gone, and she could walk using a walker and had much more mobility in her hands. When she walked around the city plaza, a few people recognized her: "Aren't you the person who was pushed around in a wheelchair a while ago?"

"Yes, it was me."

"What happened to you?" a man asked.

"I'm so lucky. I found a doctor of oriental medicine, and he gave me neuro-acupuncture treatments."

At the next session, she was excited to report her progress to me. "With the increase in my hand movements, I was able to hold a knife with both hands and cut vegetables. To be able to cook again brought me such tremendous joy and gratitude that I laughed and cried at the same time."

With each session, Julia continued to improve; however, the most dramatic changes occurred after the 20th treatment. Her leg and arm muscles had become much stronger, enabling her to write and make phone calls. So she decided to call the doctor who had the difficult conversation of giving her the dire prognosis. She said, "You told me I would be paralyzed for the rest of my life. It's not true, I can walk now."

"There is no way you are able to walk. It is hard for me to believe acupuncture could cause that to happen. I'd like to see you tomorrow, if that's OK."

The next day he went to Julia's house to see for himself this miraculous change. He was stunned as he watched her walk up to greet him. The doctor was thrilled to see her progress. He said to her, "I have many patients who need the kind of treatment you received from Dr. Hao, and I will refer them to him."

Julia had regained all movements of her hands and arms after 39 sessions and could walk safely with a cane. She finally was able to begin living without the help of personal assistants. And after 48 treatments, she felt well enough to discontinue the sessions and start a new life in the city where her son lived.

Because she didn't need the wheelchair, crutches, or cane any longer, she donated them to our clinic, just as some of our previous patients had done. That's why a sign in our office advertises: "Wheelchairs, crutches, and canes are on sale at this acupuncture clinic."

THE DISCUSSION

Often caused by car accident, spinal cord injury is extremely serious. Compression fractures due to injured cervical disks may cause permanent disabilities. Hernias or bulges of intervertebral disks may cause spinal cord compression. Common symptoms of spinal cord injuries include paralysis or weakness of the arm and leg; tingling, numbness, or pain in the affected limbs; difficulty breathing; and both bowel and urinary incontinence.

So far Western medicine has not been able to find a cure for spinal cord injury. Most of the modern methods of treatment include the use of drugs or surgery that is often unsuccessful in healing the injury or improving the symptoms. Treating patients as a whole entity, acupuncture helps those with spinal injury to regain their body's functioning more effectively than Western medical solutions. Some people with spinal cord injury are able to recover all functioning, especially those who have attained partial recovery. When all bodily functions return—motor control, bladder and bowel control, and touch and pain sensations—the recovery is considered comprehensive. While some patients can be cured through acupuncture treatment, a higher percentage experience improvement.

The best therapy for spinal cord damage is neuro-acupuncture. Proven effective through the results of clinical studies recorded over the last 50 years, scalp acupuncture is excellent at stimulating the paralyzed area by restoring the body's energy flow to a normal state, allowing the body to heal itself. In other words, neuro-acupuncture treats the cause—the diminished flow of energy—and thus heals the injury. It is by far the most efficacious technique for helping patients improve quickly in initial sessions. To ensure the best results, practitioners familiar with neuro-acupuncture will combine it with the more commonly known body acupuncture.

Electrical acupuncture may be helpful in speeding up recovery from spinal injury. Electrical stimulation usually lasts 10 to 20 minutes and can be applied on points in the limbs, as well as at *Huatuojiaji* points on the back. The pair of *Huatuojiaji* points to stimulate should be one above and one below the spinal injury site. For the recovery of affected limbs, active and passive exercises are vital. Regular exercise not only keeps muscles active, but improves blood circulation and accelerates the results from ongoing acupuncture treatments.

Q&A

How quickly does a paralyzed person get a positive response from neuro-acupuncture?

In my practice 50% of patients with paralysis receive positive responses during the first neuro-acupuncture treatment; 85% show improvement within the initial three treatments; and sessions will be discontinued after 5–6 neuro-acupuncture treatments if the patient does not show any improvement.

How do you evaluate the progress of a paralyzed patient?

Aside from the obvious physical improvements demonstrated or related by the patient, there are scientific methods for assessing progress. In neuro-acupuncture, the diagnosis, examinations, assessments, and evaluations are mostly based on neuroanatomy, neurology, and neuroscience. I apply the four diagnostic methods used in Chinese medicine—observation, auscultation (listening to the sounds of organs such as the heart and lungs), olfaction (utilizing the sense of smell), and palpation (applying pressure of the hand or fingers to the body, especially to take the patient's pulse)—for choosing Chinese herbs and determining the prognosis. Examining the tongue and feeling the pulse are the most important among the four diagnostic methods in my practice.

NOTES

Chapter Two

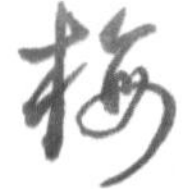

APHASIA

"It is inspiring to carry the hope for patients
who may not realize what is possible with
brain plasticity and acupuncture."

—Jason Jishun Hao, DOM

Aphasia:
The Condition and Definition

Aphasia is a neurological disorder caused by damage to the areas of the brain responsible for language. The main symptoms include difficulty in expressing oneself when speaking, in understanding others' speech, and in reading and writing. The most common cause is a stroke, but it can also manifest from a head injury, a brain tumor or infection, Parkinson's disease, or dementia that damages the brain. A stroke or head injury can bring on aphasia suddenly, while a brain tumor can cause it to develop slowly.

THE DIAGNOSIS

Aphasia has been categorized into four types: expressive, receptive, anomic, and global aphasia. The precise location and extent of the damaged areas of the brain determine the type and severity of the language dysfunction.

Expressive aphasia is caused by damage to the anterior parts of the brain known as Broca's area. This type of aphasia is also referred to as Broca's aphasia, motor aphasia, and nonfluent aphasia. People with this aphasia have the common problem of agrammatism, or the inability to use words grammatically in a sequence, resulting in speech that is a challenge to initiate, nonfluent, labored, and halting. Patients with extreme cases may not be able to utter any words at all.

Receptive aphasia is often caused by damage to the superior temporal gyrus known as Wernicke's area. It is also referred to as Wernicke's aphasia, sensory aphasia, or fluent aphasia. In this aphasia, patients often fail to make sense of spoken or written language and cannot comprehend words when they hear or see them.

People with *anomic aphasia*, or nominal aphasia, may see something but aren't able to name what it is. They have difficulty relating to words grammatically or semantically, or they may have a general naming difficulty.

In *global aphasia*, patients have experienced damage to wide areas of the language centers in the brain. They have extreme communication disabilities and may be terribly constrained in their capacity to speak or understand language.

Modern medicine has no treatment for aphasia itself, but typically focuses on the cause, such as prescribing tPA (a medication that dissolves blood clots) for acute stroke, or surgery for brain tumor, which may result in minimizing the disability to a degree.

*"Thank you so much for this miracle, Doctor.
I'm so glad I can now speak again."*

THE STORY

THE PATIENT

When 80-year-old Maria came to me for neuro-acupuncture treatment, she had been totally paralyzed on her left side ever since her first stroke six years before. Her daughter told me that, in addition to the paralysis, Maria frequently experienced severe spasms and pain in her left limbs that made her scream.

When I examined her, Maria's mind was clear, and she could understand the questions I was asking her. But when she responded, she could only make unintelligible sounds. It was clear that she had motor aphasia. Her left arm and leg exhibited no movements, and they were stiff and tight, barely able to be moved by another person. I observed that her tongue was red with a little coating, and her pulses were wiry and thready.

THE CHALLENGE

Given the considerable variability of aphasia, the effect of the treatment is difficult to forecast. Younger patients and those who have less severe brain damage are able to recover more quickly and completely. Also factored into the prognosis is the location of damage.

Imaging methods such as PET (positron emission tomography), CT (computed tomography), MRI (magnetic resonance imaging), and fMRI (functional magnetic resonance imaging) aid in defining brain function, identifying the degree of brain damage, and predicting the severity of the aphasia. These kinds of new technologies can determine the structures of the brain used for speaking and listening. Comprehensive testing of the language capacity of patients with different types of aphasia and various aphasic symptoms leads to more fruitful treatment strategies.

Treatment in many cases is especially challenging because the patients cannot speak clearly about their condition and what they are experiencing. Practitioners need to have not only exceptional techniques of gentle insertion and stimulation of the needles, but good communication skills.

THE RECOVERY

I was encouraged by Maria's positive response to her first treatment. After I inserted the needles into her scalp, the spasms, stiffness, and tightness of her left limbs improved immediately. The limbs loosened, and her daughter could move them up and down with relative ease.

I asked her what her name was. To her astonishment, she answered, "Maria."

"How old are you?"

"Eighty."

Maria's eyes filled with tears as she answered question after question with a strong, clear voice.

"Thank you so much for this miracle, Doctor. I'm so glad I can now speak again."

A short time later she was able to move her left limbs. She could pull and push her left leg with such strength that I was motivated to ask, "Would you like to try walking?"

"Yes, I would like to try," she said in a clear voice.

With the help of my assistant, she stood and walked back and forth, repeating, "Thank you so much for this miracle."

Maria built up her strength and showed improvements at each session. By the fifth treatment, she asked, "When can I get rid of this wheelchair? I hate it."

"Just be patient. You are not quite ready now, but you may be able to get rid of it within a few more treatments."

By the eighth session, she was delighted to report her progress. "Dr. Hao, I can move my left arm and hand any way I want. I got rid of my wheelchair and walk with a walker now."

By the 12th treatment, she was extremely happy. "Doctor, I don't need a walker anymore. I can move around my house by myself."

Maria recovered completely after 16 sessions. By then she was able to have a normal life and follow a routine on her own without any difficulty walking and talking. At that final session I told her she no longer needed any further treatments. She began crying and refused to end them. She said, "I need to keep coming to this clinic for the rest of my life to continue having tune-ups. I don't want the paralysis and aphasia to come back again."

The Discussion

Patients with all types of aphasia get fairly good results through scalp acupuncture. But patients with expressive aphasia tend to recover more quickly than those with other types of aphasia. Several patients treated at our clinics exhibited immediate improvement.

Family members' involvement can often be a vital aspect of treatment. Between sessions, family members need to learn how to assist their loved ones with the various exercises prescribed by the doctor to help them regain their speech functions. An effective approach during treatment is for the doctor and family members to work together and talk with the patient to distinguish subtle changes in the patient's speech function.

Most of the aphasia patients who come to our clinics fall into the expressive category of the disorder. They have had a stroke in which there was an interruption of blood flow to the brain's language areas, causing serious damage or death to brain cells. In addition to the aphasia, these stroke patients often have other disorders, including paralysis, altered coordination, difficulty swallowing, and mental and emotional changes.

We have found that scalp acupuncture has an excellent result with expressive aphasia, with the potential for full functional recovery. As soon as the aphasia patient's condition becomes stable following a stroke, it is wise to seek acupuncture treatment immediately for the best outcome—the earlier, the better. Many aphasia patients treated at our clinics experience significant improvements at the first session, while most show some improvements within the first three treatments.

Regular acupuncture treatment involving several types of techniques has a positive effect on recovery from expressive aphasia. Scalp acupuncture has the best and fastest response, but combining it with other needling techniques enhances its effectiveness. Depending on the individual situation, a patient can be treated with body acupuncture, electric acupuncture, and moxibustion along with scalp acupuncture to quicken the recovery time.

Electrical stimulation is a viable alternative to rotating the scalp needle. For older or weaker patients, moxibustion can boost the efficacy of scalp acupuncture. Because of scalp acupuncture's excellent results, it should be the main technique, not a complementary technique, for treating patients with expressive aphasia.

Q &A

What is the average number of neuro-acupuncture sessions I might expect for aphasia?

It depends on the disease or condition causing the aphasia, the patient's history of disorder, and the patient's physical condition and motivation to follow the doctor's recommended health-related actions apart from acupuncture treatments. Generally speaking, it takes 3–15 treatments, with an average of 7–8 treatments.

For what kinds of aphasia will the prognosis be better?

According to my 40 years of experience with neuro-acupuncture treatments, expressive aphasia has the best response and recovers quicker than other types of aphasia. Receptive aphasia is next, nominal aphasia is a little more challenging, and global aphasia is the most difficult to recover from.

NOTES

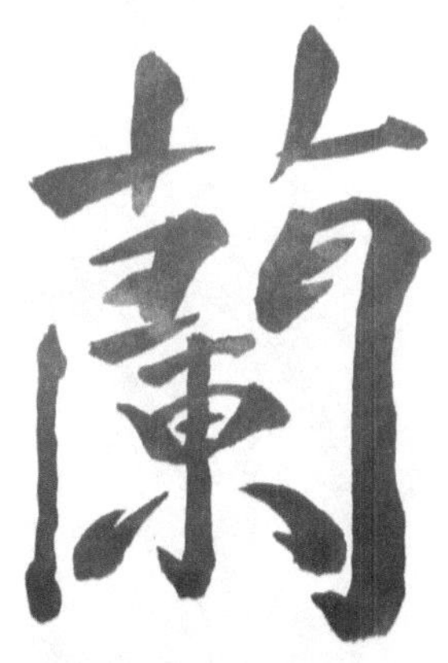

PART TWO

ORCHID

"I alone cannot change the world,
but I can cast a stone across the water
to create many ripples."

—MOTHER TERESA

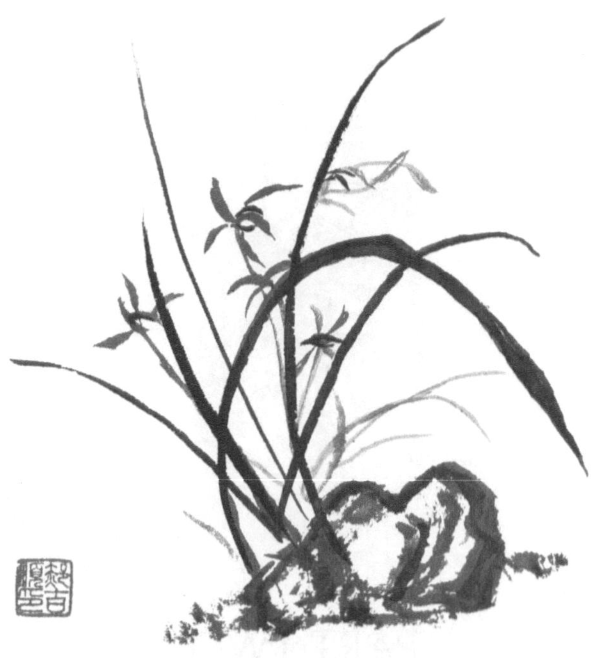

Representing spring, a season that offers new growth, the orchid has been cherished for centuries in China for its beauty and grace. Its delicate nature, elegance, and mild fragrance symbolize nobility and humility.

My Story: Graduation Ceremony at the Neuro-Acupuncture Institute

It was late spring heading toward summer in Santa Fe and the roses were just beginning to bloom everywhere. Their refreshing and delightful fragrance wafting in the air has been ingrained in the fullness of my memory and experience. It made me think of the unique blooms of people's souls, as balance comes from each petal perfectly spiraled from their heart center.

On May 1, 2019, 78 neuro-acupuncture students from the United States and around the world successfully completed the advanced course and examinations. They earned the certificate of completion for becoming proficient in the special techniques of neuro-acupuncture and were the first graduates of the Neuro-Acupuncture Institute in Santa Fe, the institute I founded and still serve as president. At the post-ceremony celebration, I delivered my speech with tears in my eyes. I was filled with joy that after 40 years of hard work in China and America, my efforts had finally paid off. I was harvesting the fruit of my labors in Chinese acupuncture.

Dressed in white lab coats with the emblem of the Neuro-Acupuncture Institute, the graduates reported on their two years of learning and clinical practice, sharing the details of their many successful cases. Their faces glowed with satisfaction from all they had learned, with confidence in the skills they had mastered, and with the joy that comes from being able to help patients recover from their disorders. Many graduates excitedly related how they could now successfully achieve the same curative effects as the professors, earning tears of relief and joy from the patients and families who benefited from their treatments.

We had invited extraordinary experts from all over the world and the United States to teach the advanced course. These professors' teaching methods and medical skills generated supreme confidence in the students. My wife, Dr. Linda Hao, and I demonstrated advanced neuro-acupuncture needling skills. Dr. Daniel

Jiao offered classes in Chinese medicinal herbs to prescribe for patients. Dr. Li Erqiang taught advanced techniques of needle manipulation. Dr. Yang Guanhu detailed his practice and experience in the treatment of diabetes and its peripheral neuropathy. Dr. He Yuxin revealed his "secret" method of treating anxiety disorders. Dr. Poney Chiang from Canada demonstrated a new therapy for peripheral nerve stimulation. Dr. Richard Skurla superbly analyzed brain neuroanatomy according to Western medicine. Dr. Sunil Pai explained a comprehensive therapy for inflammatory diseases. The entire teaching and learning experience proved to be rich and profound for all.

The demonstration of actual case treatments was the highlight and essence of the entire training course. During neuro-acupuncture treatments, three autistic children significantly improved their concentration, attention, and speech. The tremors of a Parkinson's patient stopped immediately. The balance of patients with multiple sclerosis became normal. Patients with congenital defects of eyesight had clear vision. The vertigo of a patient with brain injury disappeared. A patient with aphasia due to the aftereffects of stroke was able to speak clearly.

I treated a 19-year-old woman with cerebral palsy who then exhibited better balance, speech, and standing. Her mother started to cry when she saw her daughter move her left arm over her head for the first time in her life. Her daughter was able to open and close her left hand, also for the first time. Her slurred speech improved, and she walked for the first time without a cane.

The training program of the Neuro-Acupuncture Institute (NAI) is divided into three levels: primary, middle, and high, lasting a total of two years. The graduation of these 78 students in 2019 was a successful milestone in the history of continuing education in traditional Chinese medicine in Western countries. It received much attention in news reports and interviews.

With the intention of teaching and choosing the blessing of promoting human health, I and the other teachers at NAI passed on the wealth of knowledge we had accumulated over many years. At the end of the training, the students offered flowers, applause, and singing to give thanks to the teachers. The successful treatment cases shared by the students in their practice were the best affirmation of their newfound expertise and the return for their hard work. As I said in my speech to the graduates, "Clinical practice has proven that neuro-acupuncture has great potential for development in the West. Neuro-acupuncture can transform life and benefit mankind." The motto of our Neuro-Acupuncture Institute best explains what we are attempting to gain from our program: "The success of students is our harvest. The NAI students' successes are our achievements!"

Professor Daniel Jiao, vice chairman of the Board of Commissioners of the National Certification Commission for Acupuncture and Oriental Medicine, had kind words to say about my work and efforts: "Dr. Jason Hao is selfless and very happy to share his successful techniques. He has spent more than three years of preparation to conduct this training. Dr. Hao deserves respect for contributing this monument to the development of Chinese medicine in the United States. Congratulations!"

Chapter Three

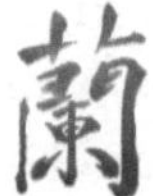

STROKE

"It's never too late to treat a paralyzed
patient with neuro-acupuncture."

—Jason Jishun Hao, DOM

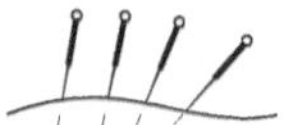

STROKE:
THE CONDITION AND DEFINITION

Stroke is an acute neurological disease in which the blood supply
to the brain is interrupted, causing brain cells to die or be seri-
ously damaged, thus impairing brain functions. This in turn can
affect the functioning of other areas of the body. Stroke is classified into two major categories: ischemic and hemorrhagic. An
ischemic stroke occurs when a blood vessel becomes obstructed
and the blood supply to part of the brain is blocked. In a hemorrhagic stroke, a blood vessel in the brain ruptures and bleeds,
interrupting the brain's blood supply to the vessel's target tissue.

THE DIAGNOSIS

The symptoms of stroke depend on the type of stroke and the affected areas of the brain. They can include weakness, paralysis or abnormal sensations in limbs or face, aphasia, altered vision, problems with hearing, taste, or smell, vertigo, disequilibrium, altered coordination, difficulty swallowing, and mental and emotional changes. At the onset of a stroke, some patients may experience loss of consciousness, headache, and vomiting. If the symptoms disappear within several minutes up to no more than 24 hours, the diagnosis is transient ischemic attack (TIA)—a mini or brief stroke. A mini stroke is a warning sign, and a significant percentage of patients with TIA have full strokes in the future.

"He was so surprised that he could move his arm and hand with just two needles on his head during his first neuro-acupuncture treatment."

—A STROKE PATIENT AT A NEW YORK TRAINING FROM 1992

THE STORY

THE PATIENT

I conducted a workshop at an acupuncture college in New York City in the early 1990s. A patient had volunteered for scalp acupuncture. The manager at the college told me the patient had a stroke from cerebral thrombosis only 11 months before and was an excellent candidate for the workshop demonstration.

I asked the patient, "What is your name?"

"Tom."

"What is your major complaint today?"

"My right arm and hand are paralyzed from a stroke."

"How long have you had this problem?"

"Eleven years."

"Excuse me, how long ago did you have a stroke?" I asked the question in another way to confirm the length of time he had his condition.

"Eleven years," he repeated.

When I asked Tom these questions, the doctors were shocked to find that his right arm and hand had actually been paralyzed for 11 years, not 11 months. I was a little nervous hearing this too because we had just taught their students that, generally speaking, a patient with paralysis for more than three years has no chance of recovery by acupuncture.

"What do we do about him? Do we still treat him?" one doctor asked me with a low voice in Chinese. "It took several hours for his wife to drive him here. We really cannot say no to him. He will be very disappointed."

"Well," I said, "let's do it like this. We will only demonstrate the location and technique of neuro-acupuncture. We will not show the result for this patient."

After the doctor put two needles in the scalp of the patient, she took him to another room and inserted some more needles.

THE CHALLENGE

Stroke is a major cause of death in the United States, behind only heart attack and cancer, and it is one of the leading causes of disability in adults. With standard modern medical treatment, stroke patients need immediate attention. The earlier the stroke is diagnosed and treated, the more likely the patient will survive and have less severe symptoms. These symptoms depend on the affected area of the brain and the degree of brain tissue damage. About 75% of stroke survivors have some form of disability that often includes one or more physical, mental, or emotional disorders.

Stroke patients need to begin rehabilitation as soon as possible after the acute stage of the stroke to help them regain such functions as speaking or walking. The modalities include acupuncture, massage, physical and occupational therapy, and speech therapy.

THE RECOVERY

While Tom and his wife, Diane, were in another room, she was instructed to give him some passive exercise by moving his hand

and raising his arm. As we continued the lecture, we heard a scream coming from that room.

Tom and Diane rushed back into the lecture hall. In a loud, excited voice, Diane said repeatedly, "He can move his arm and hand now." Tom demonstrated by moving his arm, hand, and even his fingers in any way the audience asked him to.

"What do you think about this?" I asked the audience. "It's incredible. I wouldn't have believed it if I hadn't seen it with my own eyes."

The other doctor said, "Me too. Now I have to change the information I gave you a few hours ago. Patients with paralysis should be treated no matter how long ago they had a stroke, as long as their limbs show no muscular atrophy."

One student offered a conclusion: "It's never too late to treat a paralyzed patient with neuro-acupuncture."

The Discussion

Neuro-acupuncture has had excellent results in treating the side effects of stroke, including hemiplegia (as in Tom's case), aphasia, and abnormal sensations in the limbs. Through advanced research and brain imaging technology, we are continuing to gain greater knowledge about the extraordinary adaptability of the brain and how it can regain its ability to function after a stroke. Normal brain cells can undergo changes not only in shape; they can take on the functions of nearby damaged cells. Neuro-acupuncture takes advantage of these abilities and can either stimulate and restore affected brain tissue, or retrain the adjacent healthy tissue to compensate for the lost functions of damaged tissue.

Fortunately for Tom, his hemiplegia was caused by cerebral thrombosis, a blood clot in a cerebral artery, which has a better chance of recovery from stroke than cerebral embolism (obstruction of a blood vessel by a foreign object) or hemorrhage. I need to emphasize how highly unusual it is for a patient with a cause and symptom similar to Tom's to recover completely from only one neuro-acupuncture treatment. It can often take several weeks to several months for stroke patients to improve and recover, if at all.

Timing is crucial. As is often the case, the earlier the patient gets treatment, the better the chance for recovery. For strokes caused by thrombosis or embolism, scalp acupuncture treatments should begin as soon as practicable. For hemorrhagic stroke, the patient's condition should be stable before acupuncture is applied, around one month after the stroke. As shown in Tom's case, disabilities can be treated any length of time following the stroke, but the best response occurs within a year. The improvement tends to be more gradual the more that time has elapsed since the stroke. With long-term conditions, expectations need to be realistic, especially when a patient with paralysis also has muscular atrophy and inflexible joints.

Several acupuncture procedures are included in the treatment of stroke-induced paralysis. Scalp acupuncture provides the best and fastest response, but other techniques are beneficial for a fuller recovery. Depending on each patient's condition, regular body acupuncture, electric acupuncture, and moxibustion, as well as physical therapy and massage, can enhance scalp acupuncture to quicken recovery. Regular acupuncture treatment on limbs has had positive effects on regaining movement of hands, fingers, feet, and toes.

A substantial number of clinical studies and papers on experimental research show the superb results of scalp acupuncture on stroke-induced paralysis. Jiao Shunfa, the founder of scalp acupuncture, analyzed 20,923 cases of paralysis caused by stroke from 1970 to 1992 that were treated on the motor area of the scalp. After treatment, 7,637 cases were cured (36.5%), 7,117 showed marked improvement (34%), and 5,196 cases showed some improvement (24.8%)—a total effective rate of 95.35%.[2]

Jia Huai-yu reported similar results on 1,800 cases treated by scalp acupuncture in 1992. The results: 462 patients fully recovered (25.67%), 950 markedly improved (52.78%), 292 improved (16.22%), 96 failed to improve (5.33%)—a total effective rate of 94.67%.[3]

Q&A

How soon can a stroke patient get neuro-acupuncture treatment?

It depends on what type of stroke a patient suffers from. Those patients who had an ischemic stroke due to cerebral thrombosis or cerebral embolism should receive neuro-acupuncture treatments as soon as possible after the stroke. Patients who had a hemorrhagic stroke should not get treatment until their condition becomes stable. Generally speaking, these patients begin receiving neuro-acupuncture sessions one month after their stroke.

How quickly can a stroke patient see a result?

In my practice, most of the patients show some improvement within the first three treatments. About 60% of patients see results after their first treatment for paralysis, aphasia, or loss of balance. The more motivated the patients are to follow any other prescribed treatments, such as exercise, physical or occupational therapy, or massage, the quicker their improvement.

NOTES

Chapter Four

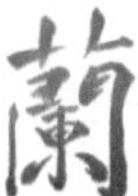

MULTIPLE SCLEROSIS

"It's incredible. I wouldn't have believed that neuro-
acupuncture could make a quadriplegic patient
walk again with just two treatments if
I hadn't seen it with my own eyes."

—A MEDICAL STUDENT AT A PHOENIX SEMINAR

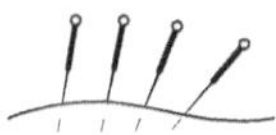

MULTIPLE SCLEROSIS:
THE CONDITION AND DEFINITION

Multiple sclerosis (MS) is a progressive disease of the central nervous system that causes a disruption in the electrochemical messages between the brain and other parts of the body. The effects vary from relatively benign for most patients, to the extreme of being totally disabling and devastating for others. During an MS attack, inflammation occurs in the white matter of the central nervous system in random patches called plaques, followed by the destruction of myelin. Myelin enables the smooth, high-speed transmission of electrochemical signals between the brain, the spinal cord, and the rest of the body. Damaged myelin can result in these neurological transmissions being slowed or blocked completely, causing some bodily functions to decline or be lost completely. [4]

A 2019 study funded by the National Multiple Sclerosis Society found that nearly 1 million people over 18 in the US suffer from MS.[5] The number worldwide is more than 2.3 million. It primarily affects adults, beginning between the ages of 20 and 40 years, and is two to three times more common in women than men.

Multiple sclerosis is unpredictable. It may occur in separate attacks or develop slowly over time. Bodily functions may recover completely between attacks, but neurological issues tend to persist, especially as the disease progresses. Though many factors have been found that increase the chances of developing MS, no specific cause has been identified. It probably involves a combination of environmental and genetic factors. Western medicine has no cure for multiple sclerosis, but several treatment modalities, including acupuncture, can be used to minimize the effects of the symptoms and even bring about remission. The most practiced alternative or complementary methods are diet and nutrition (88.3%), acupuncture (86.7%), herbal medicine (81.7%), massage (78.3%), and homeopathy (73.3%).[6]

THE DIAGNOSIS

The wide variety of symptoms and signs of multiple sclerosis are determined by the location of damaged myelin sheaths. The most common symptoms of MS are weakness and spasticity in one or more limbs (50% of patients); numbness, tingling, and fatigue (40%); partial or complete blindness, blurred or double vision (31%); urinary incontinence and bowel dysfunction (17.5%); pain (15%); and reduced cognitive functioning or behavioral problems, and sexual dysfunction (10%).[7] Other symptoms include tremor, unsteady gait, dizziness, muscle stiffness, paralysis, slurred speech, and depression. The worst cases include being unable to write, speak, or walk.

"You should open a drive-through acupuncture clinic so that we don't have to walk to your clinic to receive needle insertions."

THE STORY

THE PATIENT

Denise, a 79-year-old in a wheelchair, had suffered from multiple sclerosis for more than 25 years. Her initial symptom was numbness in her right arm, which later went down both her legs. After she was first diagnosed with MS, Denise had repeated relapses and remissions with bouts of lower extremity weakness, muscle stiffness and spasms, urinary incontinence, loss of balance, and fatigue that usually lasted a few weeks to several months.

Several years ago, she had a significant decline, losing strength and sensation in both legs and leaving her unable to stand up. For a few years prior to acupuncture treatment, she was unable to stand or walk by herself because of imbalance and weakness. Denise also endured numbness, tingling, and spasms in her legs, along with urinary incontinence and extreme fatigue. My initial examination revealed that she had partial paralysis of the lower left leg that was more pronounced than that of the right. Her tongue was purple with a thin white coating; her pulses were wiry and thready, and weak pulses were also noticed in the kidneys.

THE CHALLENGE

The beneficial effects of neuro-acupuncture treatments for progressive diseases like multiple sclerosis, Parkinson's, and ALS can sometimes be temporary. Because these effects may last for only hours, days, weeks, or months, ongoing neuro-acupuncture treatments are necessary. Improved movement is often permanent in patients treated with scalp acupuncture for stroke- or trauma-induced paralysis, but that's not the case for patients with paralysis caused by MS. As is often the situation with neurological disorders, scalp acupuncture should be considered the primary method of treatment for the patient with multiple sclerosis, rather than being complementary to other modalities.

THE RECOVERY

Denise responded well to her first scalp acupuncture treatment. She was amazed to feel the spasms and numbness in her legs improve just minutes after a few needles were inserted in her scalp.

"My leg spasms are much better, Doctor. I can't believe I could improve so quickly."

She was suspicious and nervous when I asked her to stand up. She said, "No, I can't." But, with my encouragement, she tried and was able to stand. Her family was thrilled to see she was not only able to stand up with improved stability and balance, but she also could walk a few steps.

When she arrived for her second treatment, Denise said, "My incontinence has improved remarkably, and the numbness, spasms, and weakness of my legs has improved even more." She continued to get better with each additional treatment. By the sixth treatment, Denise no longer needed to enter our clinic in a wheelchair, but came in using a walker instead. She also felt more energized and had started to do some housework again.

By the 15th treatment, Denise was happy to let me know she was able to walk around her house by herself and walk longer distances. She had more energy, and the numbness and tingling in her limbs had decreased to a point where they no longer bothered her as much. And her incontinence hadn't been a problem for several weeks. But her right foot was still weak, and sometimes it was difficult for her to pick it up, so she had to drag it when she walked. During each ensuing treatment, however, her right foot continued to get stronger and she could pick it up more easily. This ability would last for several days after treatment, so Denise liked to get a tune-up treatment every other week. At each session, I inserted a few needles in her scalp, and then she would go out for a walk and come back later for me to withdraw the needles.

Denise witnessed many of my patients who also had difficulty walking go through the same routine treatments as hers, so she came up with a suggestion for me: "You should open a drive-through acupuncture clinic. That would save a lot of time for both you and your patients. They could stick their heads out their car window to be inserted with a few needles, and then drive back through thirty minutes later to have their needles removed." What a clever idea to consider for the future!

THE DISCUSSION

Scalp acupuncture has been shown to have better results in treating MS and other central nerve damage than acupuncture on the ear and other areas of the body. It not only diminishes the symptoms, improves the patient's quality of life, and slows the progression of MS toward disability, but it can decrease the number of relapses. As with other neurological disorders, the earlier the patient gets treatment, the better the chance of recovery. Scalp acupuncture treatment for MS has had excellent success in reducing numbness and pain, decreasing the number and intensity of spasms, and improving balance as well as weakness and paralysis of limbs. In addition, many patients have reported significant improvement in their bladder and bowel control, fatigue, and overall sense of well-being.

Recent studies have shown that neuro-acupuncture can be a highly effective modality in controlling MS. As in Denise's case, neuro-acupuncture can frequently produce extraordinary results after just a few needles are inserted in the scalp. Symptoms are often relieved immediately, and remarkable outcomes are sometimes achieved in a matter of several minutes. Scalp acupuncture areas are chosen based on the patient's particular symptoms. The primary acupuncture areas for patients with MS symptoms such as paralysis and weakness of limbs or abnormal sensations in limbs, including tingling, numbness, or pain, are the motor area and the sensory and foot motor areas. Many patients have had a quick positive response in controlling urinary and bowel functions when the foot motor and sensory areas are stimulated.

Although there certainly are other acupuncture techniques that can be efficacious, scalp acupuncture is a more effective modality in bringing about quicker and often immediate improvements. When combined with regular body acupuncture and other Chinese and Western healing modalities, scalp acupuncture's effectiveness can be increased. For example, regular body acupuncture in combination with scalp acupuncture has been shown to have a positive effect on the MS patient's recovery of movement and reduction of abnormal sensations of the hands, fingers, feet, and toes.

In a clinical study at our National Healthcare Center in Albuquerque, we treated 16 MS patients using scalp acupuncture. After only one treatment per patient, 8 of the 16 patients instantly showed significant improvement, 6 patients showed some improvement, and only 2 patients showed no improvement—a total effective rate of 88%.

Q &A

What multiple sclerosis symptoms tend to improve first when the patient starts neuro-acupuncture treatment?

Most patients with multiple sclerosis have many symptoms—the typical nature of the disease. In the first acupuncture session, patients usually experience improvements in their balance, paralysis, rigid limbs, and urinary incontinence. For patients experiencing fatigue, double or blurred vision, and tingling and numbness of limbs, it often takes a few treatments.

Of the patients you've treated, who has had the longest history with multiple sclerosis and still attained a good result?

I treated a patient who had multiple sclerosis for more than thirty years and she still had good responses. Of course, the shorter the history of MS a patient has, the quicker recovery that person usually achieves.

NOTES

"Why is this miraculous form of neuro-acupuncture still not available coast to coast in the US?"

THE STORY

The Patient

Charles, a 58-year-old lawyer who came to our clinic in Albuquerque, had been diagnosed with multiple sclerosis 20 years earlier and was currently only able to work part time. His initial symptoms were numbness in the right arm followed by numbness descending both legs. From the beginning of his diagnosis, Charles had experienced multiple relapses with incidents of lower extremity weakness, stiffness and muscle spasm, urinary incontinence, imbalance, double vision, and fatigue. These symptoms usually lasted a few weeks to several months.

About eight years into his diagnosis, he had a dramatic neurological decline and was unable to walk steadily and lost strength and sensation in his lower extremities. Over the three years leading up to his visit to the clinic, it had become even more difficult for him to walk due to weakness in his legs and imbalance. Charles also had numbness, tingling, and spasms in his legs, accompanied by urinary incontinence, double vision, poor memory and concentration, dizziness and vertigo, heat intolerance, and severe fatigue.

Several MRIs showing lesions in the brain and spine had confirmed his diagnosis. Family history revealed that a brother with MS had died in 1999, and two sisters had been diagnosed with MS.

During the first neuro-acupuncture session, I conducted general and neurological examinations. Charles was awake, alert, cooperative, and attentive and gave appropriate responses. His motor strength was a 4 out 5 in both legs and 5 out of 5 in both arms and in his hand grip. Charles could not make rapid movements with the toes of either foot. My examination revealed no sensory deficit in either his face or his four extremities. His finger-to-nose tests on both right and left sides were abnormal, as was his index finger–to–index finger test. Charles had difficulty getting out of a chair and walked with a spastic and uncoordinated gait, with stiffness in both legs, unsteadiness, and a wide-based stance. He failed the heel-toe walking test and could not stand on one leg. He was also unable to stand steadily with eyes open and performed even worse with eyes closed.

During my Chinese medical examination, his tongue was red and slightly purple with a thin yellow coating. His pulse on the left side was wiry and rolling; on the right side, it was wiry and thready, and weak pulses were also noticed in the kidney positions. When I palpated points, LR-3 (*Taichong*), GB-34 (*Yanglingguan*), UB-18 (*Ganshu*), and SP-9 (*Yinlingquan*) were very tender and resulted in sharp pain, and UB-23 (*Shenshu*) and UB-15 (*Xinshu*) were tender and showed dull soreness.

THE CHALLENGE

Most healthcare practitioners in the West are familiar with acupuncture for pain management. However, a relatively new concept is applying scalp acupuncture as a useful tool for the treatment of MS. So little is known about this kind of treatment that it is not surprising for a Western physician to assert that it is a coincidence or natural remission when a patient recovers from MS after a series of acupuncture sessions. Yet neuro-acupuncture can offer solutions in circumstances where modern Western medical treatments are limited at best. It provides an excellent opportunity to expand treatment options for MS in both conventional and complementary or integrative therapies. Not only can it improve patients' symptoms and quality of life and slow and reverse the progression of physical disabilities, but it can decrease the frequency and number of relapses and help them stay in remission.

The Recovery

Charles had an excellent response to his initial neuro-acupuncture treatment. Just minutes after a few needles were inserted in his scalp, he was amazed to feel an improvement in his dizziness, balance, stiffness, and weakness in his legs. He was initially suspicious and nervous when I asked him to stand up with his eyes closed. Not only was he able to stand up with improved stability, but he could walk much more easily.

His wife was excited and teary-eyed when she observed what was happening during his first treatment. She said, "Charles, your body was very stable and didn't swing to the side at all when you were standing up with both eyes closed."

At the second treatment, Charles reported that he no longer had urinary incontinence, and the numbness, spasms, and weakness in both legs showed some improvement too. He continued to get better with each ensuing treatment. By the third treatment, Charles's vision had significantly improved, and he no longer experienced double vision and heat intolerance. He also had more energy and was able to get more done at his law office. By the fifth treatment, Charles was able to walk around his home and office without any problem and could walk much longer distances. The numbness and tingling in his limbs did not bother him anymore. His energy had increased further, and he continued to be able to hold his urine.

During the 10th neuro-acupuncture session, I conducted general and neurological examinations again. Charles was awake, alert, cooperative, attentive, and gave quicker responses. Motor strength increased to a 5 out of 5 in both legs, and remained at that level for both arms and hand grip. Unlike the initial examination, he was able to make rapid movements of the toes on both feet. I noticed no sensory deficit in his face and four extremities. Charles's finger-to-nose tests on both right and left sides returned to normal, as did his index finger–to–index finger test. He got out of a chair without any difficulty and walked with a normal gait. He performed the heel-toe walking test with no problem and could stand on either his left or right leg steadily. He was also steady when he stood with his eyes open or closed.

During my Chinese medical examination at this 10th session, his tongue had changed to slightly red with a thin white coating. His pulses changed to soft on both left and right sides, and pulses in the kidney positions changed to thready. When I palpated points, all the previous sensitive ones were neither tender nor painful and sore.

After the 10th treatment, Charles was able to work full time and started to take vacations again. He said he enjoyed standing on one leg during work breaks just to feel like a normal person. I felt confident that he now needed only one treatment a month. When Charles had a routine eye examination, his eye doctor said, "I have practiced more than 40 years and have never seen any eye problem that recovered like yours. It's hard to believe that acupuncture could do such effective work. Please keep getting treatments."

Although Charles returned to a normal life and has had no relapse of multiple sclerosis for 13 years since he started neuro-acupuncture treatments, he prefers to come to the clinic every four to six weeks for maintenance.

CHARLES'S TESTIMONY

You are likely to wonder, "What is a longtime local lawyer doing writing about serious medical problems like multiple sclerosis and Parkinson's disease?" It is because I have had the rare opportunity of taking part in what I unhesitatingly tell everyone is nothing less than a miracle. What was uppermost was that 20 years earlier I had been diagnosed with multiple sclerosis—one of the great remaining medical mysteries. MS took my brother in 1999 and has crippled one of my sisters and compromised the life of my youngest sister.

I had managed to keep the disease under control and under wraps by wisely following my wife's advice on nutrition, exercise, and a commonsense approach to MS. Together we made trips to leading medical centers where I became a voluntary "guinea pig" for new medications. On top of that, I was tested, scanned, poked, and prodded over and again by some of the best neurologists and medical professionals studying the disease.

Finally, despite all that, the symptoms were taking their toll, especially in the heat of the Mesilla Valley's long summer. I realized I could no longer continue as head of the law firm I had helped to build over three decades. When my firm dissolved, I joined another law firm on a part-time basis to comply with limited energy and "finish up" my days as a lawyer.

So, on a hot July day I awaited my first client at my new office, never anticipating that he would lead to a miracle. That client was Dr. Vittal Pai, whom I'd known for more than 20 years. I had not seen him in a couple of years and always enjoyed visiting with him. Dr. Pai, an ear, nose, and throat specialist, is a brilliant doctor known as much for his philosophical approach to life and his quick thinking and wit as he is for his substantial skills as a physician. He observed my condition and placed a card on my desk, saying, "Before we talk business, you must go see this doctor." I looked at the card and saw the name Dr. Jason Hao, Doctor of Oriental Medicine and Acupuncture.

After exchanging greetings, I told Dr. Pai that I had been a subject in medical studies at universities with the best neurologists in the world. Other than steroids, I was disqualified from all the medications that had been approved to combat MS. Those of you who know Dr. Pai also know his serene smile. He looked at me and said, "You must go see this doctor. I cannot explain how this works. I can only tell you that I have seen the results." He told me about a patient with Parkinson's disease who had incurable tremors that could not be controlled by medication. He told me that after treatments with Dr. Hao, the tremors had gone away. He told me about another patient with mobility damage from a stroke who seemed to have been miraculously cured with Dr. Hao's technique. I took Dr Hao's card, and the miracle began.

As I write this testimony, I have had 12 treatments so far with Dr. Hao at his clinic in Albuquerque, New Mexico. He practices a little-known acupuncture technique called "neuro-acupuncture." That's right, he puts needles in my head. Not only does he put needles in my head, but he spins these needles with his fingers between 200 and 400 times a minute. Dr. Hao told me that all of the nerves in the body can be accessed in the scalp and that the spinning of the needles clears the nerve pathways that have become broken and clogged. The treatments last about an hour and are relatively inexpensive and completely painless.

After these treatments, all of my major symptoms of MS are gone. My left foot, which had been numb for 18 years, is no longer numb. The fatigue that has bedeviled me as well as the heat intolerance are gone! My vision has improved, my balance has returned, and I have not had vertigo in some time. Every aspect of my life is better. I am working full-time again, although Dr. Hao cautions me that MS is still my greatest enemy and that he has only relieved me of the symptoms brought on by the attacks. He cautions me to never use more than 70% of my energy in any 24-hour period and to take the prescribed herbs and follow basic nutritional guides.

My wife and I look at each other on a daily basis and expect for this dream to end: this dream about a Chinese doctor in Albuquerque who spins acupuncture needles in my head to make the symptoms of MS go away. But every day I feel better, and my treatments with Dr. Hao are now on a monthly basis rather than a weekly basis. My energy is back. Twenty years of debilitating symptoms that compromised every aspect of my life reduced to a memory in six months! Those who knew me before last July and see me now at first just can't believe their own eyes.

In view of my changes and my many inquiries to Dr. Hao, I cannot help but wonder: Why is this miraculous form of neuro-acupuncture still not embraced coast to coast in the US?

THE DISCUSSION

Charles's case shows that scalp acupuncture is a more effective modality in bringing about quicker and often highly effective improvements to patients with MS compared to any remedies that modern Western medicine offers. Chinese scalp acupuncture is also more easily accessible, costs less, entails less risk, can yield quicker responses, and usually causes fewer side effects than some other treatments.

Though many hypotheses and research reports on scalp acupuncture for central nervous system disorders and pain management have appeared in Western medical literature over the past 50 years, modern medicine still has a long way to go in uncovering the mystery of how scalp acupuncture works. Future study is needed to investigate the mechanisms underlying acupuncture's effect on dysfunctions of the central nervous system in patients with MS. If it becomes more widely applied, we will not only be able to learn more about the mystery of scalp acupuncture, but it will become better known as a viable treatment, resulting in a significant impact on recovery from central nervous system disorders for thousands of patients. There is a pressing need for Chinese scalp acupuncture to be studied and perfected using modern research methods so that its potential can be fully explored and applied.

Q &A

Does a patient with multiple sclerosis need to continue treatment indefinitely?

Most patients with multiple sclerosis have some setbacks, unfortunately, and need to continue neuro-acupuncture treatments after they go into remission and have no symptoms. Some other neurological disorders, such as stroke or cerebral palsy, do not require the patient to continue treatments after recovery.

How often do those patients need treatment?

After an initial series of frequent acupuncture sessions, they usually receive treatments once every month or two, or every other week depending on the individual patient's condition. Some elderly patients like to get treatments once a week to continue feeling better overall and also to be able to maintain their current level of physical activities.

NOTES

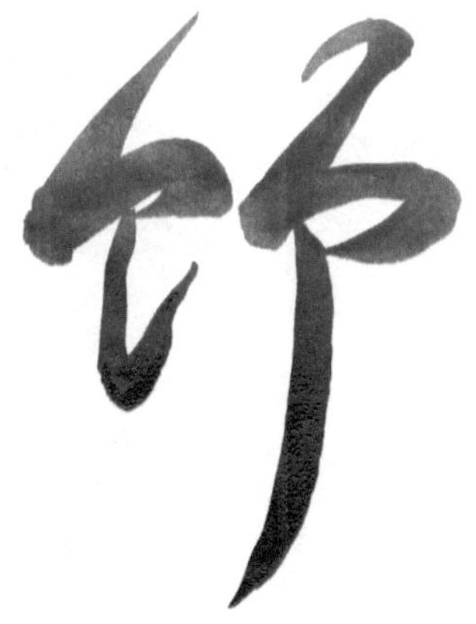

PART THREE

Bamboo

"The most beautiful experience we can have is the
mysterious. It is the fundamental emotion that stands
at the cradle of true art and true science."

—Albert Einstein

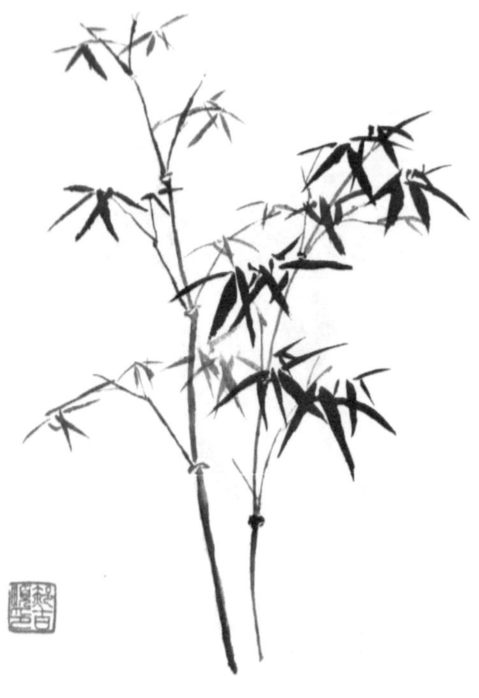

The bamboo depicts summer. Its stalk is hollow, representing open-mindedness and tolerance. It is also strong and flexible, a symbol of cultivation, integrity, and strength—values that allow one to yield when wisdom dictates that response, yet remain unbreakable. Bamboo also characterizes elegance.

My Story: The Film Premiere

As high mountains stood out against a beautiful blue New Mexico sky, yellow arnica wildflowers were dancing with Shasta daisies everywhere—as if to celebrate a big film event on neuro-acupuncture. The wildflowers of the high desert adapt and grow where they find their natural healing power in sunlight.

A new documentary by Doug Dearth, director of the award-winning documentary *9000 Needles*, premiered on May 7, 2021, at an international Zoom event at a music studio in Santa Fe. *Return to Life* highlights the Neuro-Acupuncture Institute and the efforts of my wife, Linda, and me to disseminate the groundbreaking therapy for neurological disorders that has transformed the lives of countless people. Through interviews with us, Western medical practitioners, and patients who have benefited from neuro-acupuncture, *Return to Life* documents the life-changing results this technique has had on debilitating neurological diseases, including stroke, spinal cord injury, post-traumatic stress disorder, multiple sclerosis, cerebral palsy, and autism.

Speakers at the virtual premiere included Binsheng Sang, secretary general of the World Federation of Chinese Medicine Societies; Mina Larson, CEO for the National Certification Commission for Acupuncture and Oriental Medicine (NCCAOM); and Javier Gonzales, former mayor of Santa Fe and late vice president and chief development officer of the Christus St. Vincent Foundation. "The film *Return to Life* shows us how acupuncture cooperates with modern medicine to achieve excellent results in the treatment of many neuro systems diseases," Sang said.

"The work that's showcased in this film really demonstrates how individuals with debilitating illnesses are brought back to life, and the NCCAOM is committed to promoting this and really working together with the Neuro-Acupuncture Institute to let every single American be able to do this," Mina Larson, the CEO of NCCAOM said.

At the film's core are stories shared by patients and family members who have benefited from neuro-acupuncture. Some outstanding stories include that of the multiple sclerosis patient covered earlier who regained his vision and balance, a spinal cord injury patient given a one percent chance of walking again celebrating his ability to use a walker, a mother's reaction to hearing her child with spinocerebellar ataxia and autism speak for the first time, and a veteran diagnosed with traumatic brain injury and PTSD who was freed from night terrors and pain.

The video also chronicles the Neuro-Acupuncture Institute's efforts to train more doctors and practitioners in this life-changing and often lifesaving procedure. "My mission with this film is to inspire the public with hope," I said at the premiere. "Families and their loved ones suffering from difficult neurological disorders don't have to suffer the rest of their lives. With just a few needles we can reduce the burden from these diseases. We want to transform their life, change their life, and help them to return to life. If this pandemic has taught us anything, it is that we are all in this world together, and we need to help each other."

Chapter Five

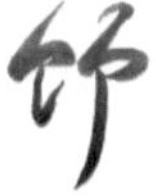

CEREBRAL PALSY

"With just a few needles we can reduce the burden on the body by opening pathways that can lead a patient toward natural healing, and transformation in order to return to life."

—JASON JISHUN HAO, DOM

CEREBRAL PALSY: THE CONDITION AND DEFINITION

Cerebral palsy (CP) is a group of disorders that affects a person's mobility and balance and is caused by damage to the motor centers of the brain, manifesting as a lack of muscular coordination and as speech disorders. It may occur in children in utero, during childbirth, or after birth up to about the age of three.[8] Most children with cerebral palsy have it at birth, though it may not be detected until months or years later. The brain damage is often caused by genetic abnormalities, stroke, maternal infections and fevers, or fetal injury including stroke in utero. United Cerebral Palsy's fact sheet states that an estimated 764,000 children and adults in the United States are living with one or more symptoms of cerebral palsy.[9] According to the Centers for Disease Control and Prevention, about 10,000 infants born in the United States each year will develop cerebral palsy.[10] The incidence of dysarthria—a CP-related disorder in which speech muscles are dysfunctional—is estimated to range from 31% to 88%.[11]

THE DIAGNOSIS

Historically, Western medicine has believed that damage from cerebral palsy is irreparable and the resulting disabilities are permanent. The diagnosis relies on the patient's history and physical examination. Once a child is diagnosed with cerebral palsy, no additional diagnostic tests are needed. CP tends to require a lifelong multidimensional process of treatment focused on overcoming developmental disabilities or learning how to accomplish challenging tasks in new ways.

*"I won second place at my school's swimming race
and enjoy playing the drum at my school."*

THE STORY

The Patient

Michael, a six-year-old with cerebral palsy, came from Texas with his parents to the Neuro-Acupuncture Institute in Albuquerque several years ago. His mother gave me details about his condition, reporting that he had barely any coordination of the muscles in his upper and lower extremities and had never spoken a sentence they could understand. Michael was unable to write or draw anything with a pencil because his hands were too weak to make even a mark on the page. For two years he had been passive in kindergarten due to his inability to write, speak, or participate in physical activities. He made little effort to communicate. Owing to his low level of functioning, he had initially been diagnosed with mental retardation and learned helplessness. Multiple medical doctors, including neurologists and ear, nose, and throat specialists, evaluated Michael and the most likely diagnosis was that he had suffered a stroke in utero.

Michael had been receiving speech therapy and physical therapy for several years with no noticeable improvement.

My examination showed no abnormality in his physical development or hearing. It was difficult to understand him when he spoke his name, age, and birthday or when he counted.

His coordination was severely impacted. He couldn't touch his nose, bring his index fingers together, or kick his legs. His tongue was red with a thin white coating, and his pulses were wiry and slippery.

THE CHALLENGE

Cerebral palsy affects more than 17 million people worldwide.[12] CP is the most common motor disability in childhood, and in 2003 the Centers for Disease Control and Prevention estimated that the lifetime cost of care per individual can amount to $1 million.[13]

Western medicine has been mostly ineffective in the treatment of CP. This means that hundreds of thousands of cerebral palsy patients in the US are without adequate solutions for their condition. However, the patients treated at our clinics show the effectiveness of Chinese scalp acupuncture in improving the symptoms of CP. Neuro-acupuncture is accessible and cost effective, with no adverse side effects to date. When treatment is successful, the response rate tends to be rapid.

For most healthcare practitioners familiar with acupuncture for pain management, scalp acupuncture as a useful tool for the treatment of CP is a new concept. Chinese scalp acupuncture may be able to provide solutions in situations where Western medicine is limited, and with further, much-needed research and experimentation, it holds the potential to increase the number and efficacy of treatment options for patients with CP and other central nervous system disorders.

THE RECOVERY

Michael was a bit nervous about having needles put in his head during his first treatment. He seemed to understand that the needles would help him become a normal kid, and he was able to keep his body still when I inserted the needles. I noticed that he moved his head slightly during one needle insertion, so I asked him with kind voice, "Did this needle hurt, Michael?"

"No," he replied with strong voice.

"Do you feel better?" I asked after I adjusted the needle a bit.

"Yes, sir."

He was so glad to hear himself speak better during and at the end of his first treatment. It was easier to understand him when I asked him again what his name and age were. When he counted from one to ten, most of the numbers were clearer after the treatment than they were beforehand.

During the second session, Michael had little fear of the needle insertions. He tried hard to pronounce clear sounds and make everyone around him excited. He attempted to repeat the words and sentences his parents and I were saying, and he succeeded in speaking many of the words clearly so that we could understand them. He seemed very happy when he discovered he was able to kick his legs and stand on one leg without difficulty.

When they arrived for the third session, his mother reported that Michael had started to talk in clearer sentences, some of which she could understand completely. And that morning he had succeeded in dressing himself by the time she went to wake him up to come to the acupuncture clinic.

During the fourth treatment, Michael was able to speak almost like a normal child, sing a song clearly, and laugh. By the fifth session, his parents said he was more physically active and had even less trouble speaking. His fear and anxiety both at school and at home had diminished. Michael was playing with other children and, based on his teacher's report, had made some improvements in his schoolwork. When I conducted an examination, I found that he could speak more clearly and write or paint like a normal child. His physical activities, such as jumping, kicking, running, and standing on one leg, showed no restriction at all. The redness of his tongue was now only on the tip. I decided he could start coming for treatments every other week instead of once a week.

Following the 10th session, Michael's speech and grades in school, as well as speech and physical activities at home, had significantly improved. However, he still had trouble saying certain words, particularly those beginning with *s* or *r*, such as *school, stop, rabbit,* or *rock.*

After his 14th session, Michael had become a happy, communicative, and physically active boy who could say clearly whatever thoughts or feelings he wanted to express, and move his body and limbs as he wished. His mental and physical activities were no longer restricted. His parents happily reported that his math and reading scores had progressed by a grade level, and he was advanced to first grade.

His grandparents brought Michael to see me for a checkup once a year for eight years. After five years it was apparent that Michael had become a normal boy in both mental and physical activities. He was delighted to give me this report: "I won second place at my school's swimming race and enjoy playing the drum at my school." A remarkable testimony to his excellent coordination.

Our final examination showed that his tongue was a little red with a thin white coating, and his pulses were soft. His case study was accepted and published immediately after I submitted it to the journal *Global Advances in Health and Medicine.*

The Discussion

The scalp somatotopic system—the relation between particular areas of the body and the corresponding motor areas of the brain—seems to operate as a miniature transmitter-receiver in contact with the central nervous system and endocrine system. By stimulating those reflex areas, acupuncture appears to have a direct effect on the cerebral cortex, cerebellum, and other areas of the brain. The scalp's unique neurologic and endocrinal composition makes it an ideal external stimulating field for the internal activities of the brain.

Scalp acupuncture has had significant success in treating cerebral palsy and to not only improve symptoms and the patient's quality of life but to reverse mental and physical disability and restore normal brain function. We have used scalp acupuncture to treat children with a variety of CP symptoms, including paralysis, ataxia (lack of coordination of muscular movements), hypotonia (deficient tone or tension) or hypertonia (excessive tone or tension), apraxia (inability to perform coordinated movements), dysarthria (trouble speaking), dysphasia (inability to use or understand language), and mental retardation. Advanced brain research and imaging technology have enabled scientists to continue to better understand how the brain can adapt after damage and even regain its ability to function. A child's brain is not fully developed until about the age of eight, and has the plasticity to be able to reorganize, adapt, and reroute signals if it is stimulated properly. In addition, brain cells not only can change in function and shape but take over the functions of nearby damaged cells. Because of these inherent capabilities of brain cells, scalp acupuncture can apparently stimulate and facilitate the recovery of affected brain tissue and support the retraining of unaffected brain cells to compensate for the lost functions of the damaged tissue.

I have found that verbal communication with children and their parents during treatment helps to reduce their fear and anxiety. It is often important to encourage a child with aphasia to talk, count, or sing in order to exercise the power of speech.

During treatment, some patients may have some or all of the following sensations: hot, cold, tingling, numbness, heaviness, distension, and the sensation of water or electricity moving along their spine, legs, or arms.[14] Those sensations are normal, and patients who experience some or all of these sensations usually respond and improve more quickly. However, those who do not have such sensations may still have positive results—sometimes immediate.

The time frame for patients with cerebral palsy to be treated with scalp acupuncture is important. Parents should have their child receive acupuncture treatment as soon as his or her condition is diagnosed. Because the brain is more elastic at a young age, the earlier the child receives treatment, the better the prognosis.

Western medical science and neurology have not yet found an explanation for the success of scalp acupuncture in treating CP and other central nervous system disorders. A growing body of clinical evidence in the US and China indicates that scalp acupuncture can improve or remove symptoms in patients with cerebral palsy. Given the lack of effective treatments in conventional medicine, it is important for neuro-acupuncture to be studied and approved using modern Western science and technology. More case reports are needed to inform clinical practice and generate testable hypotheses for clinical trials so that patient care can be improved through neuro-acupuncture and its potential benefits.

Q&A

Is it safe for a child to have neuro-acupuncture treatments? How do they respond when you insert needles into their scalp?

I have practiced neuro-acupuncture for 40 years and have not had any problem treating children. I created special needling and communication techniques for them. Since I use relatively smaller and thinner needles for children, most of them do not feel the needles being inserted at all. They usually like to come back for more treatments after they start feeling better and experience other improvements.

Can a child with cerebral palsy recover completely?

Children's brains have more plasticity and change quickly if they receive the correct stimulation. I have helped a lot of children with cerebral palsy and some of them recovered completely.

Is neuro-acupuncture still effective for an adult who has had cerebral palsy since childhood?

Yes, I treated a 55-year-old woman who had cerebral palsy since birth. She had pain in her right hip, weakness in her right leg and foot, and needed to walk with a cane. After only three neuro-acupuncture treatments, all her symptoms went away and she could walk normally without using her cane. She referred many patients to our clinic after her recovery.

NOTES

Chapter Six

AUTISM

"Nearly four million children with autism and
their parents could live normal lives if we
could help just 20% of the total."

—JASON JISHUN HAO, DOM

AUTISM:
THE CONDITION AND DEFINITION

As defined in the *Diagnostic and Statistical Manual of Mental Disorders*, classic autistic disorder is a neurodevelopmental disorder characterized by difficulties with social interaction and communication, and by restricted and repetitive behavior. The signs develop gradually, and parents often begin noticing them during the first three years of their child's life.

Autism may be associated with a combination of genetic and environmental factors. How it affects information processing in the brain and how neurons and their synapses connect and organize in autism is still not clear. It affects approximately 24.8 million people worldwide as of 2015.[15] Since the 1990s the number of people diagnosed with classic autism has increased considerably, perhaps partly due to better diagnosis of the condition.

THE DIAGNOSIS

Because neither the exact cause nor the neurological mechanism of autism has been identified, diagnosis is generally based on behavior. Children with autism are usually identified by the deficiencies in their communications and interactions with others in a variety of situations, by their repetitive patterns of behavior, and by their restricted interests and activities. These deficits appear in early childhood and develop into significant impairment. Common symptoms include lack of social or emotional give-and-take, unvaried and repetitive use of language, and preoccupation with unusual objects.

"We have a new problem now. Our son has turned into a talking box after the last treatment. We cannot stop him from talking."

THE STORY

THE PATIENT

Tony, a four-year-old autistic boy with aphasia, traveled from Texas with his parents to our office in Santa Fe one summer. An acupuncturist in Texas had referred his parents to me so Tony could receive neuro-acupuncture therapy. His mother told me he had never spoken any words since birth and was having seizures every two or three weeks. His parents had taken him to many ear and throat specialists and neurologists with no clear diagnosis or explanation as to the cause of these symptoms. Several intensive examinations, including magnetic resonance imaging (MRI) and electroencephalography (EEG), didn't succeed in coming up with a diagnosis. Tony had been receiving speech therapy for one year without any positive outcome. Although he had aphasia, my examination at the clinic showed no abnormal findings of his mental activities, coordination, physical development, and hearing. His tongue showed a red tip with a thin white coating, and his pulses were slippery.

The Challenge

It has long been assumed that there is a common cause at the genetic, cognitive, and neural levels for autism's characteristic triad of symptoms: impaired communication, impaired social skills, and repetitive and restricted behaviors.

The main goals when treating autistic children are to decrease the severity of the symptoms as well as the family's distress, and to increase quality of life and functional independence. So far in conventional Western medicine, there has been no effective treatment, and any treatment implemented is typically tailored to the child's needs.

The Recovery

Though the little boy was afraid and crying before the beginning of treatment, he was quiet and cooperative during the insertion of the needles. To help him relax, I selected the ear point *Shenmen* for the first needle, which serves to reduce sensitivity to scalp acupuncture. However, he didn't even notice when I inserted the needle in his ear, showing no negative reaction at all. Next, I placed four needles on the speech I area and foot motor and sensory area of his head and left the needles there without any stimulation by rotation. He didn't exhibit any obvious improvement during and after the first treatment.

During the second session of scalp acupuncture, he was not afraid, and said to me in sign language, "I love you and thank you." He felt a little pain, but his tension was soon abated by a new toy his mother showed him as I inserted the last needle. He tried hard to make some sounds to get his favorite new toy. His mother and I lit up with pleasure.

"He is starting to have a positive response now," I said.

"We have really prayed for this for a long time," she responded.

Tony attempted to repeat the conversations I was having with his parents and continued to make many kinds of sounds while he was playing with his mother and me, but no one understood what he said. Laughingly, his parents wondered if the sounds he was making could be Chinese or some other foreign language.

Prior to the third session, his mother reported that Tony had started to speak more clearly in sentences she could understand better. She also said that when she went to his room to wake him up that morning, she found him already dressed and acting anxious. "When I asked him what was the matter, he said, 'I want to see that doctor.'"

At the fourth session, the treatment room was filled with laughter and excited chatter because Tony was speaking like a normal child. At the beginning of the fifth treatment, his mother smiled and said, "We have a new problem now. Our son has turned into a talking box after the last treatment. We cannot stop him from talking." His mother added, "He got up early and was anxious to see you again this morning." The little boy and I were laughing and talking a lot during this treatment. He even had a series of questions for me: "Are you Chinese, Doctor?... How old are you?... Do you have a kid?... What is his name?"

At the end of the fifth session, I told his parents that this was the last treatment Tony needed, and his mother replied, "He will probably feel sad when he hears he doesn't need to see you anymore." As they were leaving, Tony's mother said to the little boy, "Now what do you say?" He responded, "Thank you very much, Doctor. Good-bye." Then there were hugs all around.

At a consultation three months after his final treatment, his parents reported that Tony was still speaking like a normal child, and that he had not experienced any more seizures. How relieved and grateful we all were!

THE DISCUSSION

Language disorders affect children and adults differently. For children who do not use language from birth, the disorder often occurs in the context of a language not fully developed or acquired. An adult with aphasia may hear or see a word but not be able to understand its meaning, and they may have difficulty and frustration trying to get others to understand what they are trying to communicate.

An infant is initially able to make controlled sound as the vocal mechanism matures, and this manifests in the first few months with cooing. By six months, an infant usually babbles or repeats simple syllables such as *ma ma,* and *pa pa.* Babbling then takes on the rhythm of speech but is still unintelligible. Mastery of a few words usually comes after a year, and by 18 months most children can say 8 to 10 words. Two-year-olds can begin saying short "sentences" by combining a few words together and begin expanding their vocabulary with words for objects, actions, and thoughts. After age two, children's language ability progresses rapidly.

If parents have concerns about their child's speech or language development, they should discuss it with their child's pediatrician or a speech pathologist before the child reaches age five, which is also the age limit when a child with aphasia since birth has a better chance to respond well from scalp acupuncture.

Q &A

What is your best result for a child with autism from neuro-acupuncture treatments?

I treated a 16-year-old boy with autism during a lecture in Dubai a few years ago. He had been unable to talk and communicate with other people since he was two years old. During his first neuro-acupuncture treatment at my class, he was able to speak a few words, then some phrases, and finally some sentences. He was overjoyed to be able to talk with me.

Can autistic children improve other symptoms besides speech?

Yes, most children with autism show improvements in their behaviors, emotions, activities, and concentration during and after their neuro-acupuncture treatments.

NOTES

Chapter Seven

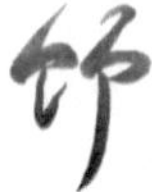

TRAUMATIC BRAIN INJURY

"The documentary film *Return to Life* traces my
wife, Linda, and my journey as DOMs [Doctors
of Oriental Medicine] who are developing and
documenting a unique integrated healthcare approach
that is rethinking and discovering acupuncture's
new role in today's modern medicine."

—Jason Jishun Hao, DOM

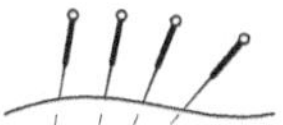

Traumatic Brain Injury: The Condition and Definition

Traumatic brain injury (TBI) is a serious condition that may lead to permanent or temporary impairment of the brain's functions. Brain damage is often related to a forceful impact on the head, resulting in injury to the corresponding area of the brain as well as its opposite area. A traumatic brain injury may also include damage to the scalp and skull. The symptoms depend on the affected areas of the brain and the functions those areas perform. For example, when speech and motor areas are damaged, disorders such as aphasia and paralysis result. The most common causes of TBI in the US include car accidents, violence, construction injuries, and sports and recreational injuries. Motorcycle and bicycle accidents are becoming more prominent causes in developing countries. An estimated 1.6 to 3.8 million traumatic brain injuries each year in the US have been the result of injuries from sports and recreational activities.[16]

Brain injuries can often be prevented by using seat belts in cars and helmets when riding bicycles and motorcycles, and implementing fall prevention methods for older adults and various safety measures for children.

DIAGNOSIS

Because the brain provides the body and mind with so many functions, TBI can result in a wide variety of symptoms—besides the many relating to just physical and cognitive functions—such as social, emotional, and behavioral symptoms. The consequences from traumatic brain injury range from full or partial recovery to permanent disability or death. Diagnosis frequently depends on imaging technology such as computed tomography (CT) and magnetic resonance imaging (MRI).

Symptoms depend not only on the part of the brain affected but on the severity of TBI, whether mild, moderate, or extreme. Immediately after the injury, a person with mild TBI may lose consciousness up to a few minutes. Physical symptoms of mild TBI include headache, nausea, vomiting, reduced coordination, dizziness, lightheadedness, imbalance, blurred vision, tinnitus, fatigue, and insomnia. Cognitive and emotional symptoms include changes in behavior or mood, confusion, memory issues, and difficulty concentrating or thinking.

In addition to the symptoms appearing with mild TBI, a person with moderate or severe TBI may experience constant headache, frequent vomiting or nausea, convulsions, inability to awaken from sleep, pupil dilation, slurred speech and other speech issues, weak or numb limbs, paralysis, restlessness, or agitation. Common long-term symptoms of moderate to severe TBI include cognitive changes, inappropriate social behavior, severe emotional issues, and poor social judgment.

"Thank you very much. Our family is very happy to see her riding her bicycle again."

THE STORY

THE PATIENT

When ten-year-old Lisa's primary care doctor recommended neuro-acupuncture treatment, her mother brought her to our Santa Fe clinic in a wheelchair. Four months earlier, Lisa had fallen off her bicycle and hit her head above and behind her left ear, resulting in a concussion on the left side of the brain. Initially she was completely paralyzed on her right side and unable to speak. After starting physical therapy, osteopathic therapy, and speech therapy two weeks after her injury, her aphasia gradually improved, and she was able to drag her right leg while walking and move her right arm slightly. But her paralysis had not improved in the eight weeks prior to her arrival at our clinic. When I examined Lisa, her tongue was red with a thin white coating, and her pulse was rolling and wiry.

THE CHALLENGE

Children with moderate to severe TBI may not be able to describe their symptoms, as would certainly be the case if a child has aphasia or is very young. Additional TBI symptoms seen in young children include persistent crying, inability to be comforted, lethargy, lack of interest in eating, and irritability. As with other neurological disorders, Western medicine is limited in its ability to treat the symptoms of traumatic brain injury, so most patients with moderate to severe TBI have to endure a long recovery or suffer a permanent disability. It can be challenging enough to treat children with body acupuncture, and even harder with neuro-acupuncture. Children and their parents might not be willing to participate in pediatric needling as a therapeutic method.

THE RECOVERY

Lisa was afraid of needles and started to cry and refused the treatment before I inserted the first needle. She screamed, "I don't want needles in my head! It'll hurt." She finally agreed to allow me to insert needles only after her mother told her she might be able to ride a bike again if the treatments worked. The insertion of two needles on the left side of her scalp did not seem to bother her at all.

"Did the needles hurt you?" I asked.

"I didn't feel anything."

Two minutes later Lisa said, "I feel a lot of blood moving to my head." She was then able to lift her right arm with much more ease. Her walking also improved because she was able to lift her right leg more easily.

With every visit, she experienced dramatic improvements in her right arm, hand, leg, and foot. By the sixth treatment, Lisa could move her right arm up and down quickly and was able to start writing with her right hand again. After the 15th session, her hand had increased in mobility and use and was now as strong as her left hand. Her walking appeared almost normal, and she was able to run slowly.

At the end of the 22nd treatment, her right hand was completely back to normal, and all the paralysis was gone. She was beaming when she said, "I ran in a race at school and did very well. Thank you very much for helping me, Doctor. I thought I would never run again after my injury." At Lisa's final visit, her family brought me a bouquet of beautiful flowers. The accompanying note read: "Thank you very much. Our family is very happy to see her riding her bicycle again."

THE DISCUSSION

Scalp acupuncture offers excellent rehabilitation tools for traumatic brain injury. The practitioner needs to have not only excellent techniques of insertion and manipulation of needles, but excellent communication skills, especially when treating children. Sometimes it is necessary to show a child how tiny the needles are, or demonstrate the insertion of a needle in the practitioner's own body. This helps to reduce fear and anxiety for both patient and parents.

Before treatment, it is helpful to play or chat with young patients as if they were friends or family members so they can be more relaxed. It is also a good idea to ask the parents to talk, play with, or even feed young patients during the insertion and stimulation of needles. These actions divert the child's attention away from the needles and make the young patient less sensitive to the procedure.

If a child is extremely sensitive to needles, stimulation by twirling should be avoided during the first one or two treatments. For children younger than two years old, an effective technique is to hide each needle from their sight while inserting and twirling. For the most part, children should receive fewer needles, milder stimulation, and a shorter period of needle insertion. No matter the age of the person, practitioners need to observe the patient's responses to the treatment and their reactions while inserting, stimulating, or withdrawing needles, and to adjust the techniques accordingly.

Q&A

What is the age of the youngest child you treated with neuro-acupuncture?

I treated an infant with nystagmus 20 years ago. He was 14 weeks old and his eyes had been bouncing back and forth nonstop since birth. After he recovered at nine months old, his mother was inspired to attend an acupuncture college and become an acupuncture professor and practitioner.

How many treatments on average are required for children to recover from traumatic brain injury? For adults?

Children's brains have more plasticity than adults' and are able to recover more quickly from damaged brain cells. Generally speaking, children with TBI recover after 5–10 treatments, while adults require 8–15.

Notes

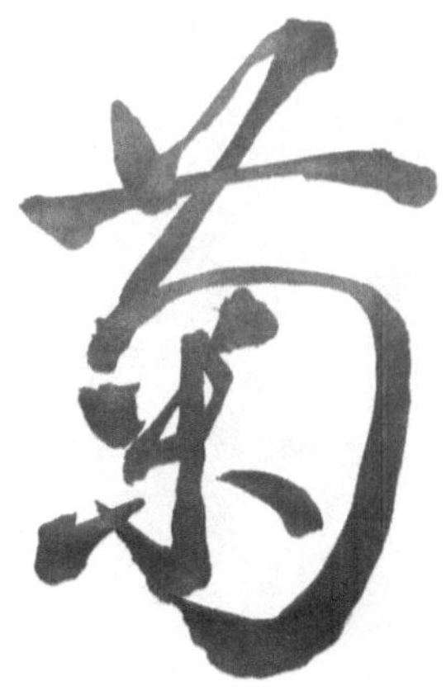

PART FOUR

CHRYSANTHEMUM

"Being deeply loved by someone gives you strength;
loving someone deeply gives you courage."

—LAO TZU

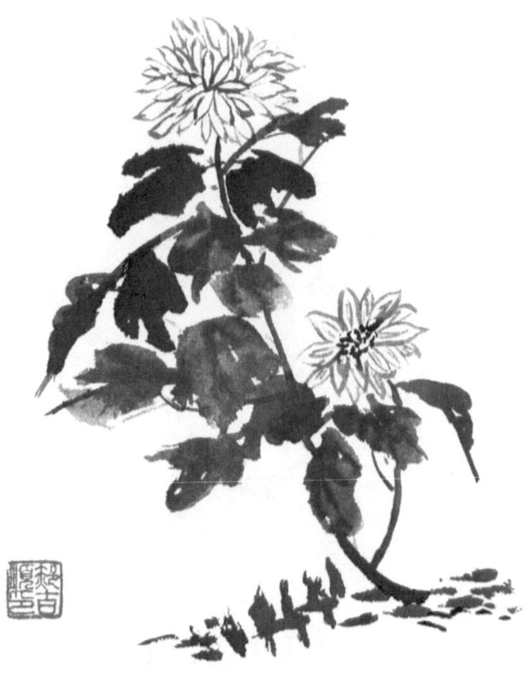

Representing the transforming season of autumn, chrysanthemums bloom later in the year, offering them little competition with countless flowers that bloom in the summer months. They give us a beautiful and elegant feeling of being at home. Some chrysanthemums bloom in the cool temperatures of autumn and are harbingers of the coming of winter months, symbolizing the ability to withstand any approaching adversities.

MY STORY: LECTURE AT WALTER REED NATIONAL MILITARY MEDICAL CENTER

On the morning of February 11, 2006, in the state of Maryland, a heavy snowstorm became so thick that the fir trees outside our hotel room almost disappeared. There was excitement to begin our first day teaching and demonstrating scalp acupuncture at Walter Reed Medical Center. In that frozen world, as the beautiful snow decorated the pine trees, the storm tipped the balance of my emotions from adventure to caution.

Because of the snowstorm, the seminar was delayed two hours. My mind was very much unsettled and challenged because it was the first time in my professional life to present neuro-acupuncture to military physicians from the Army, Navy, and Air Force, showing them how this technique could alleviate phantom pain. In addition, I had been told that all five demonstrations of ear acupuncture treatments by another doctor had failed during a presentation the previous day.

At that time in 2006, there were several hundred veterans at Walter Reed who had lost their limbs during the wars in Iraq and Afghanistan and who suffered from phantom pain. The physicians at the center tried to help them with all kinds of conventional treatments but had only limited results. Walter Reed medical leaders started to look for better solutions by considering alternative medicine. Through research, they discovered that acupuncture could have good results in relieving pain and even phantom pain.

I was invited to Walter Reed to demonstrate and teach neuro-acupuncture treatments for phantom pain, complex regional pain, and residual limb pain. Attendees were physicians from various Army sections at Walter Reed and Brooke Army Medical Center, as well as several doctors from the Navy and Air Force. Following hours of lecture in the classroom, the course participants and I visited injured service members on Ward 57.

I performed neuro-acupuncture treatment on several eager patients who had severe phantom pain. After only one treatment per patient, three of the seven patients instantly felt relief, showing significant improvement and reporting no pain (43%). Three patients showed some improvement (43%), and only one patient showed no improvement (14%), yielding a total effective rate of 86%.

"Acupuncture can help reduce pain so that fewer or lower pain medications would be needed and patients can more quickly progress to higher levels of physical functioning," said Col. Jeff Gambel, MD, chief of the Walter Reed Amputee Clinic and course coordinator. He presented me with an award at the end of the course.

Following the instruction and demonstration, Col. Gambel said, "All course participants were grateful to Dr. Hao, who made it possible for them to further explore acupuncture as one alternative approach to better help our nation's heroes during their recovery."

Walter Reed Medical Center's newspaper, *Stripe,* reported our success in a story on the front page titled "Easing the Pain" on February 17, 2006. The article gave a highly favorable report about acupuncture for the treatment of pain, and it resulted in a positive impact on spreading the practice of acupuncture in the West.

Many medical experts reasoned that acupuncture must work very well for pain management if physicians in the US military have learned it. Since then, I have been invited to a number of countries to conduct acupuncture seminars, and have given many lectures at international conferences.

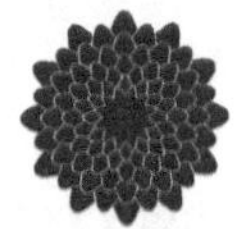

Chapter Eight

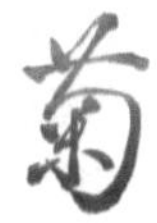

PAIN

"All course participants were grateful to Dr. Hao, who made it possible for them to further explore acupuncture as one alternative approach to better help our nation's heroes during their recovery"

—Col. Gambel, MD
Chief of the Walter Reed Amputee Clinic

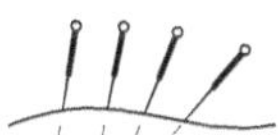

Pain:
The Condition and Definition

Pain is defined by the International Association for the Study of Pain as "an unpleasant sensory and emotional experience associated with, or resembling that associated with, actual or potential tissue damage." It is the most compelling motive for patients to visit doctors' offices in most developed countries and is often a significant symptom in many physical disorders. Pain is often referred to using such terms as severity, its acute or chronic nature, location, and cause. The most common classifications of pain are acute pain, which occurs suddenly and lasts a relatively short period of time, such as a sprained ankle, and chronic pain that lasts for several months and perhaps years, such as chronic plantar fasciitis.

Depending on the characteristics of any given pain—its severity, longevity, and location—it can have a major influence in a person's ability to function normally without any limitations. For example, people with significant pain in one or both feet could be limited in their ability to stand, walk, run, drive, and dance for long periods. Depending on the cause of foot pain, a smooth and easy recovery may be hard to come by with Western medicine.

THE DIAGNOSIS

Plantar fasciitis is typically diagnosed by a doctor who performs a physical examination and takes into consideration a patient's medical history and risk factors. The inner heel bone on the sole may be painful to the touch. Extreme tightness of the Achilles tendon or the calf muscles may cause the foot to have limited ability to flex upward, which will tend to cause pain from the stretching of the plantar fascia. Because of the ability to diagnose plantar fasciitis through physical examination, imaging methods such as X-rays and MRIs are not usually needed for diagnosis but may sometimes be used to exclude the possibility of more serious causes.

The heel pain associated with plantar fasciitis tends to be sharp and often most intense when putting weight on the heel after getting out from bed in the morning or after sitting for a long period. The pain often improves as the person continues walking following a rest period.

"Doctor, I thought I would end up sitting in a wheelchair for the rest of my life because of my heel pain. It doesn't bother me anymore."

THE STORY

THE PATIENT

Lucy, a 53-year-old teacher, came to our Santa Fe clinic for severe heel pain. My son, David, observed how painful it was for his teacher to stand and teach and had suggested that she come to our clinic. At the time, David had been in the US for only a few months and knew just a little English and Spanish.

He said, "Ms. M, you need to see my dad for your feet."

"What does your dad do?"

David couldn't say "acupuncture" in English yet. So instead, he said, "You will feel better after he puts many, many needles in your feet."

Lucy guessed that I must be an acupuncture doctor. She had been diagnosed with plantar fasciitis a year before. When she came to see me, I told her that acupuncture is highly effective for relieving heel pain, but sometimes the insertion of needles around the heel can hurt due to inflammation of the nerve endings. She had a strong desire for relief but no interest in surgery, so that made her a willing patient for acupuncture.

Lucy had burning and stabbing pain in the bottom of her left heel and in the entire bottom area of her right foot. Her feet were painful in the morning and became further exacerbated as the day progressed in the classroom. She had tried other treatments, such as orthotics, steroid injections, physical therapy, and medication for inflammation, but with no lasting, positive results. When I examined her, I found that both her heels were swollen and very sensitive to touch. Her tongue was red with a little coating, her pulses were wiry and thready, and her kidney pulses were weak as well.

The Challenge

Currently, Western medicine does not offer an effective and long-lasting remedy for plantar fasciitis. Though many patients have been prescribed corticosteroid injections, the pain relief is short-lived, lasting a month or less. Opioids for pain relief bring their own serious problems, including the dangers of addiction, overdose, and death.

Patients have also tried other common methods recommended by their doctors, including anti-inflammatory medicine, rest, massage, heat, ice, and exercises to stretch and strengthen calf muscles. Alternative therapies include physical therapy, chiropractic adjustments, psychotherapy, and acupuncture. Not many patients know about neuro-acupuncture and how effective it is for plantar fasciitis. And even if they're familiar with acupuncture, they might be reluctant to try it, fearing the treatment will cause more pain.

The Recovery

During the first treatment, Lucy was extremely sensitive to the needles around her feet. However, I was able to insert all the needles for her treatment except those in the bottom of her heels. Even so, she was very happy to leave our clinic with some relief from her pain. During the second session, though I did both ear and scalp acupuncture first to reduce her sensitivity to the needles in her heels, Lucy still experienced quite a bit of pain from heel needles. When I inserted a needle in the bottom of one heel, she screamed so loudly it startled everyone in the clinic. Fortunately, she felt significant improvements after the second treatment, and she was able to stand and walk with such a lower level of pain that it was tolerable.

With each additional session, Lucy gradually experienced more improvement and less sensitivity to the needles in her heels. However, she still screamed at every session. When I hesitated to put the needles in the bottom of her heels, Lucy would insist on their insertion, saying "No pain, no gain," to encourage both me and her.

By the eighth treatment, Lucy said, "I no longer have any pain in either foot and have even been able to wear many pairs of shoes that I couldn't wear for some time." Because of neuro-acupuncture, she has been free of pain for 28 years now. At her final treatment, Lucy said, "Doctor, I thought I would end up sitting in a wheelchair for the rest of my life because of my heel pain. It doesn't bother me anymore." She was so happy that her feet were pain-free and that she didn't need any more acupuncture treatments. Lucy has been a family friend ever since my son's elementary school days.

THE DISCUSSION

Acupuncture has been used to treat a wide range of different kinds of pain for approximately 3,000 years. Over the last three decades in the West, acupuncture has gained increasing popularity in relieving pain, especially musculoskeletal pain. Acupuncture methods for pain management include acupuncture of the scalp and body, including ear, hand, and foot.

The positive results of acupuncture for relieving heel pain are due to its ability to relax the foot's connective tissue and muscles, reduce inflammation, and promote circulation of Qi and blood in the feet. Typically, the pain continues to diminish with each treatment. Patients might compensate, consciously or unconsciously, for their heel pain by standing or walking differently, which could cause additional issues or imbalances. Acupuncture is not only effective in treating heel pain, but also in balancing the whole body, benefiting the legs, hips, and low back pain.

In my practice I have found it beneficial to use other acupuncture methods in addition to scalp acupuncture to enhance the effects, including needling points on the bottom of the feet. Based on my clinical experience, electrical stimulation to the foot's local points with high frequency and low intensity is also very helpful.

Sometimes it is necessary to identify what physical and lifestyle factors may be contributing to the heel pain that may reduce the effectiveness of the acupuncture treatments, or cause the pain to return. For example, the patient might need to lose weight and limit their time spent standing or walking.

Q &A

What kinds of pain respond well to neuro-acupuncture?

I have treated a lot of patients with pain and have had good responses in the past 40 years, including those with migraines, trigeminal neuralgia, phantom pain, complex regional pain, upper and lower back pain, neck and shoulder pain, leg and foot pain, sciatic pain, and pain from shingles or post shingles.

Do you use other Chinese medical methods to treat patients with pain?

Yes, I often combine acupuncture with Chinese herbs, cupping, electronic stimulation, and moxibustion to enhance neuro-acupuncture treatments. Each method or set of methods has a specific purpose in the treatment of various circumstances and symptoms.

NOTES

Chapter Nine

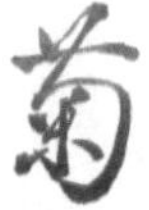

PHANTOM PAIN

"The motivation to help our wounded warriors
requires new thinking beyond conventional treatments.
Neuro-acupuncture offers promising success for our
veterans with the application of regenerative medicine."

—Physician's consensus at
Walter Reed Medical Center

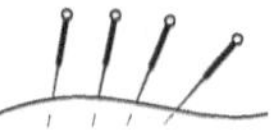

Phantom Pain:
The Condition and Definition

Phantom limb pain refers to the various types of discomfort felt in an amputated limb. Up to 80% of patients develop phantom pain post-surgery.[17] To the person with an amputated limb, the missing leg or arm gives the sensation of still being present. The pain manifests in a variety of ways: burning, squeezing, cramping, prickling, shooting, or stabbing. The cause is unknown, though several theories have been suggested. If researchers can come to an understanding of the underlying mechanisms of phantom pain, it could possibly lead to effective types of treatment.

THE DIAGNOSIS

The diagnosis of phantom limb pain is straightforward, but what isn't obvious is the cause. According to some studies, there are indications that the pain may have its origins in the brain. The area of the brain that formerly controlled the now missing limb no longer has a function, so other areas of the brain fill in. The primary sensory cortex, subcortex, and thalamus undergo reorganization after amputation. One theory considers the reorganization of the sensory cortex to be responsible for phantom pain.

Modern Western medicine has not provided an adequate solution for treating and fully eliminating this kind of pain. However, acupuncture is becoming a more promising and better-known method of treatment for phantom limb pain.

*"You can't remove the needles. They need
to stay there permanently because
they relieve my phantom pain."*

THE STORY

THE PATIENT

Rick, a 22-year-old soldier, waited his turn for a scalp acupuncture treatment at Walter Reed National Military Medical Center near Washington, DC, on February 11, 2006, when I was there to give a lecture and demonstration. Although several months had elapsed since both of his legs had been amputated, he still felt severe phantom pain. The medications the doctors prescribed offered little relief, and the pain prevented a good night's sleep and caused him to lose control of his emotions. Rick described extremely painful tingling sensations in both feet, with his right foot worse than his left. During my examination I noted that his tongue was red with a thin white coating, and his pulses were wiry and rolling.

THE CHALLENGE

Many acupuncture practitioners have little experience in treating phantom pain, and very few patients are even aware of neuro-acupuncture and how effective it is for reducing and eliminating that pain. There is an urgent need to conduct clinical trials to explore the best acupuncture protocols for treating phantom pain so its potential can be implemented widely as a viable method for eliminating the suffering these patients currently have to endure.

THE RECOVERY

Soon after I inserted needles into his scalp, Rick said, "At first I started to feel heat in both of my legs, and then a tingling and almost electric-like sensation in my big toes."

"Where is the sensation now?" I asked him as I twirled the needles in his head.

"Second toes, now all my toes."

Five minutes later, Rick said, "My pain has diminished considerably." And after ten minutes passed, he said, "Oh, my lord, my phantom pains have completely disappeared."

"You mean, you do not feel any phantom pain now?" asked a physician in the audience.

"Yes, sir. I do not feel any pain now," Rick answered.

After 30 minutes had elapsed, I prepared to remove the needles from Rick's head, but he refused to let me do so, saying, "You can't remove them. They need to stay there permanently because they relieve my phantom pain."

"The needles in your head have to be removed," I said gently.

"OK, I will let you remove those needles, but you must promise me that you will put all the needles back at same places if my pain comes back after you've taken them out."

He was astonished to report that he didn't feel any pain after I removed the needles.

Still worried his phantom pain might return sometime after the needles in his scalp were removed, Rick insisted on sitting at the back of the classroom for a while. After two hours he was convinced that the pain was gone for good, so he happily left the room.

THE DISCUSSION

Neuro-acupuncture has the advantages of being less expensive and safer, and appears to have few side effects. In addition, scalp acupuncture not only decreases or eliminates phantom limb pain, but significantly adds to our knowledge of this type of pain. By directly stimulating the central nervous system in the head, it can release neurotransmitters, hormones, or the body's natural painkilling endorphins. Neuro-acupuncture may also change bodily functions that are believed to regulate and respond to phantom pain, including blood pressure, blood flow, and body temperature.

Other recent studies have shown that scalp acupuncture could be a highly effective form of pain relief for a variety of phantom limb pains. But many more scientific trials need to be conducted to more accurately assess the efficacy of neuro-acupuncture in the treatment of phantom limb pain and to determine the best protocols to follow.

Q&A

How do patients react when they feel their phantom pain disappear?

Since conventional medicine has no effective treatment for patients with phantom pain, they are told to live with it. So when I or other neuro-acupuncture practitioners treat them, they quite often become very emotional, often with crying, at the sudden decrease or elimination of pain.

I treated a young man from England who had suffered from phantom pain in his right arm for 11 years. During the session, he burst into tears and said, "This is the first time that my brain has connected with my right arm and hand since I lost them. Immediately after you inserted the needles into my scalp, my severe tightness loosened up and I felt no pain. I can't thank you enough."

Does a patient with phantom pain need to continue neuro-acupuncture treatments after the pain is relieved?

Usually not. Most of my patients with phantom pain have permanent results and don't need further neuro-acupuncture treatment. A few of them feel the pain coming back on occasion but get better again after more treatments.

How many neuro-acupuncture treatments does a patient need?

It depends on the individual patient and the history of the disorder. For some people it may take only 2–3 treatments, and for others it may require 7–8. The average is 5–6 treatments.

NOTES

Chapter Ten

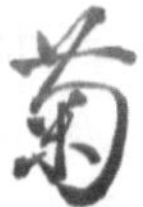

COMPLEX REGIONAL PAIN SYNDROME

"With the insertion of just a few needles, neuro-
acupuncture can bring about extraordinary results—
often immediate improvements and sometimes
in a matter of several minutes."

—JASON JISHUN HAO, DOM

COMPLEX REGIONAL PAIN SYNDROME: THE CONDITION AND DEFINITION

Complex Regional Pain Syndrome (CRPS) is a chronic pain associated with injury to an arm or leg, and yet with a severity that is frequently worse than the original injury. One type of CRPS (Type I) involves injury to skin, bone, joints, or tissues with no related nerve damage. Another form of CRPS (Type II) involves injury to major nerves. Complex regional pain may manifest in the affected area as intense burning pain along with color and temperature changes of the skin, sweating, swelling, or hypersensitivity on the injured limb. We don't know the cause or mechanism of complex regional pain; however, it often appears to be associated with a problem in the sympathetic nervous system.

THE DIAGNOSIS

There is no standard test to diagnose complex regional pain syndrome. A diagnosis of CRPS is arrived at mainly through a physical examination along with a review of the patient's medical history and current symptoms. Doctors will ask patients about their recent history, specifically any fracture, surgery, or injury, even a relatively minor one such as a sprain. In their physical examination, they will determine whether there is any change in the temperature, appearance, or texture of the skin, test for an uncharacteristic degree of pain from a given injury, or ask about any other disease or condition that could possibly be the cause of the pain, changes in skin, or other symptoms. Some physicians, especially those not familiar with CRPS, may order blood tests, bone scans, X-rays, CT scans, or MRIs to rule out other conditions that have similar symptoms.

Conventional medicine has not provided completely effective help in alleviating these types of pain. Among other alternative methods of treatment, such as transcutaneous electrical nerve stimulation (TENS), vibration therapy, biofeedback, hypnosis massage, physical therapy, and electroconvulsive therapy, acupuncture has become an increasingly popular method of treatment for acute and chronic pain.

"I haven't been able to stand or walk due to severe pain in my leg for several months now. I will make you rich if you can get me to walk again."

THE STORY

The Patient

Jeff, a 45-year-old soldier, waited anxiously for a scalp acupuncture treatment at Ward 57 while I was at Walter Reed on February 11, 2006. During a battle in Iraq, he was shot twice in each leg and now suffered from severe complex regional pain in his right leg. So sensitive were his right leg and foot that even the lightest touch or contact with a thin blanket or sock would cause severe, almost intolerable pain. Jeff could no longer stand or walk due to this sensitivity.

When I asked if he believed acupuncture could help, Jeff said, "I truly do. I've heard a lot of good things about acupuncture. From the bottom of my heart, I hope I can benefit." Then he told me, "I will make you rich if you can get me to walk again."

The Challenge

CRPS is a common and challenging condition that lacks an effective treatment in Western medicine. Unfortunately, some

CRPS patients can become extremely sensitive to any direct contact of the affected areas. This means that acupuncture, and any other modality requiring the affected area to be touched, will be extremely painful to the patient. Because of this, regular body acupuncture is not a suitable treatment in these cases. Many have reported that acupuncture near the affected area often makes the pain worse.

THE RECOVERY

As soon as I inserted the needles in his scalp, Jeff reported that he was experiencing a "water bubble–like sensation" moving first from his right hip to his leg, then to his foot and toes. Five minutes later his leg and foot pain started to diminish.

I then asked him to touch and feel his leg. He replied immediately, "I can't do it, it'll hurt a lot."

"The needles have rewired your brain, so you should be fine to touch your leg and toes."

Jeff slowly and carefully moved his hand to gently touch his leg. To his amazement he found that he could hold his leg with little discomfort. He was so excited to have such a dramatic result that he continually touched his leg and toes to verify they were indeed better. I asked him to put a sock on his right foot and he did so without any pain or discomfort. When I told him to stand up and try to walk, he experienced a lot of pain. He looked exhausted, so I ended the treatment and he took a nap. I needed to move on to my next patient anyway.

When I returned to the ward the next day, Jeff was sitting in his wheelchair with both socks and shoes on. "How has your pain been since the neuro-acupuncture treatment yesterday?"

"I've had very little pain and am much less sensitive than I was before."

"Did you walk today?"

"I didn't. I was afraid my leg pain would come back like yesterday if I tried to walk."

"You will be fine after I put needles in different places today."

When I inserted four needles in his scalp, he was able to walk with almost no pain. Each step he took brought enthusiastic applause from observers. I was eager to confirm his promise to make me rich, but Jeff replied, "I don't remember that I said that! But you are a master who knows how to cure such a difficult disorder like mine. You don't need to worry about getting rich. I have no doubt you will become very wealthy in the future."

A reporter from Walter Reed's *Stripe* newspaper observed what had happened during Jeff's second treatment. He took a photo and wrote an article titled "Easing the Pain," which was published on February 17, 2006.

THE DISCUSSION

Neuro-acupuncture has been proven to be the most effective modality for relieving pain, including those induced by central nervous system disorders. Western medical practice often opts to treat the symptoms with drugs or surgery. Neuro-acupuncture, on the other hand, has been highly effective in treating complex regional pain, phantom pain, and residual limb pain, often with remarkable results after the insertion of just a few needles in the scalp.

Other acupuncture techniques—ear acupuncture, body acupuncture, and electronic acupuncture—also have been proven effective for alleviating complex regional pain. Electronic acupuncture stimulation of ear points, *Huatuojiaji* points, and the sensory areas are all excellent places for healing complex regional pain.

Circumstances such as emotional stress, anger, fatigue, anxiety, and insomnia have been found to trigger or increase pain. Practitioners need to take this into consideration and treat each patient according to their individual symptoms and needs and select ear and body acupuncture points appropriately.

Q & A

What are your best results for treating children with complex regional pain?

When I treated a 12-year-old girl from Oklahoma with CRPS, the severe pain in her leg and foot disappeared and she was able to continue doing gymnastic performances. Her mother referred 30 children with CRPS to our clinic, and all of them recovered after five neuro-acupuncture treatments.

Why haven't more people with CRPS received neuro-acupuncture treatments given the remarkable results you have achieved?

In the past 32 years I have done my best to inform the public and the medical profession at large that neuro-acupuncture treatments are highly effective for a number of neurological conditions, including CRPS. Many newspapers and radio and television stations have reported my success stories. I can only assume that patients or their relatives believe there aren't any effective treatments for the condition and don't think to seek out alternative healing techniques such as acupuncture. They may also find it hard to believe that such a simple procedure using just a few needles can relieve excruciating pain.

I continue to train practitioners in these techniques through the Neuro-Acupuncture Institute. As more and more are trained, an increasing percentage of the public will become aware of the benefits of this extraordinary form of acupuncture.

Notes

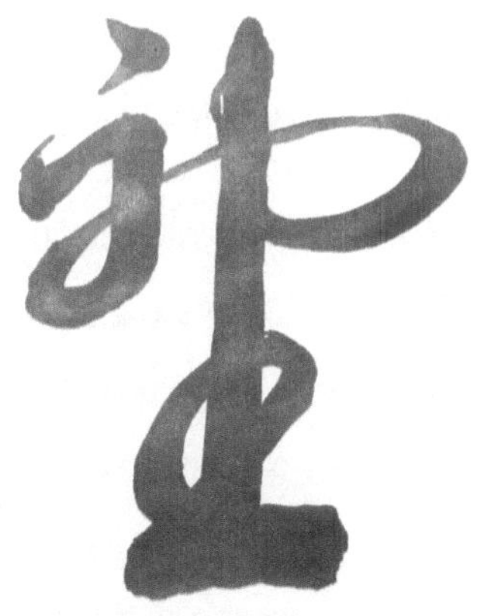

HAO NEURO-ACUPUNCTURE GIVES HOPE

"Knowledge is limited. Imagination encircles the world."

—Albert Einstein

THE FUTURE OF NEURO-ACUPUNCTURE

"The most profound development in Chinese
acupuncture in the past 50 years is the integration of
modern Western medical knowledge of neuroanatomy,
neurology, neuroscience, and neurological rehabilitation
with ancient Chinese needling methods and scalp
acupuncture to create a new technique
called neuro-acupuncture."

—JASON JISHUN HAO, DOM

HAO NEURO-ACUPUNCTURE TREATMENT FOR LONG COVID

In the past three years the COVID-19 pandemic has had a huge impact around the world on the economy, education, and especially health. According to the CDC, as of February 3, 2023, about 102,447,438 people in the United States have been infected with this coronavirus (SARS-CoV-2), and 1,106,824 people have died.[18] Globally, there have been 754,018,841 confirmed cases of COVID-19, including 6,817,478 deaths reported to the World Health Organization (WHO).[19]

Based on the latest studies, about 10–20% of those exposed to SARS-CoV-2, regardless of age or severity of original symptoms, experienced post-COVID-19 symptoms, more commonly known as long COVID symptoms.[20] WHO defines it as "the continuation or development of new symptoms three months after the initial SARS-CoV-2 infection, with these symptoms lasting for at least two months with no other explanation." Common maladies of long COVID include more than two hundred different symptoms.

Our clinical observations have found that many of its manifestations are neurological and psychiatric abnormalities. The patients mostly suffer from fatigue, anxiety, depression, irritability, brain fog, lack of concentration, memory loss, insomnia, headache, loss of taste, loss of smell, tinnitus, vision changes, shortness of breath, limb joint pain, numbness, paresthesia, vertigo, balance disorders, aphasia, limb paralysis, and a host of other symptoms.

In response to these long COVID symptoms, the entire medical community, including practitioners of traditional Chinese medicine, is facing a situation we have never experienced before, with the immediate challenge of trying to find effective treatments. After more than three years of study and practice, I have found that neuro-acupuncture has significant positive results in treating various aftereffects of COVID and also in alleviating adverse reactions to COVID vaccines.

I have used neuro-acupuncture to explore and treat various symptoms caused by the new coronavirus, and have accumulated valuable experience in treating several common symptoms: anxiety, depression, headache, loss of taste and smell, insomnia, fatigue, brain fog, dizziness, and various types of limb pain. In the use of neuro-acupuncture to alleviate the adverse reactions to the COVID vaccines, the most prominent protocol involves scalp acupuncture, including the head and foot motor sensory areas on the scalp. I have seen its miraculous effect in alleviating various neuropsychiatric symptoms, with some patients recovering after only a few treatments.

I treated a fifty-one-year-old woman from England in December 2022 who had a paralyzed left arm and foot for six months after having contracted COVID. Following two neuro-acupuncture treatments, her left arm and foot paralysis recovered, and her anxiety, depression, fatigue, and brain fog also improved significantly. She was happy with the results after the final treatment and was able to return to London.

A seventy-year-old male doctor came to me with a variety of symptoms twelve months after being infected: loss of smell, loss of taste, anxiety, fatigue, brain fog, chest tightness, and difficulty breathing. After the fifth treatment, his sense of smell and taste improved significantly, reaching 95% normal functioning. He was sleeping much better, his physical strength significantly improved, his digestion returned to normal, and he had chest tightness and shortness of breath only during exercise.

I also treated a thirty-nine-year-old male who had a severe whole-head headache immediately after his second COVID vaccine, accompanied by extreme insomnia, anxiety, and general fatigue for three months. He had taken a variety of Western medications without any relief. After only two neuro-acupuncture treatments, the patient responded quite well. The severe headache was gone, and he had no anxiety or irritability. After two weeks and three months of follow-up sessions, all the patient's symptoms disappeared, his sleep was back to normal, and he had regained his energy. He had recovered completely.

The neurological and psychiatric symptoms of long COVID and the adverse reactions of the vaccine are related to brain function, and their condition may be caused by other factors aside from the coronavirus itself, such as cerebral ischemia and the overactivation of the immune system or autoimmune reaction. In addition, reduced social contact, loneliness, incomplete recovery, and unemployment may affect psychiatric symptoms.

The mechanism leading to long COVID symptoms is still not clear. Researchers are currently focusing on four areas: blood clots and damage to small blood vessels (microclotting), immune system disorders, persistent infection with coronavirus, and impaired metabolism. Microclotting and inflammatory abnormalities might be associated with some symptoms of long COVID. They can be a result of tiny clots blocking the smallest blood vessels, capillaries, in our body. Immune system disorders related to ongoing inflammation is a normal response of the body to infection or injury, but proteins in the blood suggest that inflammation caused by COVID may cause some of the symptoms. At the same time, antibodies from the autoimmune system have been shown to adhere to human cells for a long time with the new coronavirus, causing symptoms to continue long past recovery of the initial stages of the illness. Persistent infection with coronavirus can begin in the lungs and respiratory tract, but the virus can also infect other parts of the body. Impaired metabolism is due to damaged mitochondria, which can lead to abnormalities in the body's ability to produce and consume energy.

Our clinical observations suggest that neuro-acupuncture has excellent results for the patients with long-term symptoms of COVID or adverse vaccine reactions. In Western countries, many acupuncture practitioners are familiar with acupuncture as a method of treating pain. Neuro-acupuncture not only relieves pain but provides effective treatment methods to improve, repair, and reverse the neurological, psychiatric, and other functional disorders caused by long COVID and adverse reactions to vaccines. It thus reduces the burden placed on those patients, their families, and society at large, and helps patients return to work and enjoy a normal life.

There are currently millions of people in the world struggling with a long Covid condition that affects their ability to function, to work, and to have a decent quality of life. These long-term conditions will put significant burdens on health systems worldwide for years to come. Much has to be done to overcome long COVID symptoms. I believe several important areas need to be addressed. The medical profession and the public should fully recognize the manifestation of long COVID, and no patient should be abandoned or have to struggle to navigate through a medical system that is not prepared to treat long COVID. We should gather more data, report more cases, and conduct more research and clinical trials so that through this exploration we can eventually find the best treatments for these conditions. All medical professions need to unite in order to discover effective interventions. Together, if we invest and build wholistic as well as integrative medical teams, will be able to help suffering patients.

Neuro-acupuncture has relieved many of these patients' symptoms, increased their quality of life, and reversed many of their physical disabilities. There is an urgent need for further research on the mechanism and clinical application of neuro-acupuncture so we come to an understanding of its full potential in effectively treating people with long COVID symptoms and adverse reactions to COVID vaccines. We have begun to conduct such research at the Neuro-Acupuncture Institute in Santa Fe, New Mexico, in the United States. My next book in this series will focus on my success with long COVID patients using neuro-acupuncture.

"My debilitating long COVID symptoms were relieved as soon as Jason Hao placed a few needles on my head on my first visit. I am so relieved to know I can get back to playing my guitar full time again."

—A YOUNG MUSICIAN FROM NEW YORK

EPILOGUE

Over the past 33 years, neuro-acupuncture has helped the practice of acupuncture in the United States and Europe expand into an area of medicine that was once nearly impossible to treat effectively: central nervous system disorders. The success of this dynamic component of acupuncture practice is the result of the integration of traditional Chinese needling protocols with Western medical knowledge of neuroanatomy, neurology, and neuroscience. When neuro-acupuncture is applied to patients with neurological disorders, the results are often immediate, making it clear that it is superior to other healing modalities, both Chinese and Western. It has helped many patients with a variety of medical issues, including stroke, multiple sclerosis, Parkinson's disease, traumatic brain and spinal injury, PTSD, phantom pain, complex regional pain syndrome, cerebral palsy, and autism.

In the past, there was only scant use of neuro-acupuncture among Western practitioners, mainly because of a severe lack of highly experienced teachers and the absence of an authoritative and practical text for neuro-acupuncture in English. This began to change after my wife, Linda, and I wrote and published our book *Chinese Scalp Acupuncture*, an especially valuable contribution to the advancement of acupuncture in the West. It fills a major gap in both the literature and practice of acupuncture by providing practitioners with new and highly effective techniques to treat central nervous system disorders where other therapies have failed. Since the original printing of our book in 2011, practitioners have studied and applied its principles to aid in the recovery and relief of their patients. Reprinted nine times, *Chinese Scalp Acupuncture* has been used as a textbook at many acupuncture schools in the West, and serves as the main textbook for all three course levels at our school, the Neuro-Acupuncture Institute in Santa Fe, New Mexico.

Through years of case studies and practice, significant developments in the treatment of neurological disorders have occurred since the original innovation of neuro-acupuncture a half century ago. Because of these developments, I am increasingly asked to explain the mechanisms of neuro-acupuncture. Although some research papers have focused on its mechanisms and clinical uses, the quality and quantity of research is insufficient for us to be able to adequately evaluate the results of this therapy. Even in China there are relatively few published studies that include control groups using Western standards, and many of the studies analyzed only a few changes in neurophysiology and biochemistry. In addition, the wide variety of techniques and treatment protocols applied in these studies makes it extremely difficult to evaluate the results critically. For these reasons, it is not easy to provide a logical explanation of neuro-acupuncture's effectiveness from a Western perspective.

Though we can't yet give a clear explanation of why neuro-acupuncture is so effective, it is obvious from the limited number of clinical studies, as well as my own decades of practice, that it has extraordinary results in treating central nervous system issues. In addition, some findings suggest that neuro-acupuncture improves the viscosity of the blood, improves vascular elasticity, reinforces cardiac contraction, and increases blood flow to the brain.[21]

Practitioners are continually seeking to understand what causes these successful outcomes in terms familiar to Western medicine. Currently, there are four possible explanations:

1. Neuro-acupuncture may enhance brain plasticity in promoting brain repair by stimulating the formation of new functions in the surrounding undamaged tissue.[22]

2. Circuits between neurons of the central nervous system may be able to adapt in response to external stimuli and experience.[23]

3. Neuro-acupuncture may stimulate the brain to create a new neuronal pathway or rewire a part of the damaged cortex.

4. The damaged brain can often reorganize itself such that when one part fails, other parts can compensate for it.[24]

My 40 years of extensive teaching and clinical experience have enabled me to significantly expand the variety of techniques and applications of neuro-acupuncture for the recovery of a wider range of neurological disorders. These techniques have advanced to such a degree that they provide a solid foundation for established acupuncture practitioners, as well as those new to the field, to increase their treatment options and learn how to apply them effectively and thus significantly impact their patients' lives and livelihood.

This book is the first in a series of four books that I hope will advance the continuing integration of Chinese medicine with Western medicine and herald an exciting period of increased awareness and practice of neuro-acupuncture around the world. For health practitioners who aren't using acupuncture techniques, this book may motivate them to learn and incorporate them in their practice. And of course, readers who have the medical issues discussed or mentioned in this and future books will be encouraged to seek treatment from the highly trained graduates of the Neuro-Acupuncture Institute.

In the future volumes I will introduce more cases that have been treated successfully by neuro-acupuncture. My hope is that readers of these books will benefit personally from their newfound information and share it with their doctors, families, and friends and thus help more and more people who are suffering from disorders of the central nervous system.

I see my acupuncture practice as a work in progress. Its applications are still expanding. I recently discovered that patients can recover from long COVID symptoms and adverse reactions to COVID vaccines. For example, a woman I treated who had a paralyzed left leg for three months recovered after five neuro-acupuncture treatments; a man who lost his senses of smell and taste for six months recovered after six treatments; and a man with severe headaches, anxiety, and extreme insomnia following his second vaccine recovered after only two acupuncture treatments.

There is now a pressing need for this innovative acupuncture technique to be studied and perfected using modern science and technology. With further research and the development of more effective treatments, it has great potential in enhancing the medical profession. Our increasing knowledge of neuro-acupuncture will have a significant positive impact on thousands of patients seeking relief. Fully exploring and applying this methodology will reveal its ability to return patients to a normal life.

Endnotes

(1) Brett B. McMillan, "Easing the Pain," *Stripe*, February 17, 2006

(2) Jiao Shunfa, *Head Acupuncture,* Foreign Languages Press, Beijing, 1993, p. 47

(3) Jia, Huai-yu et al., *Scalp Acupuncture Therapy,* People's Medical Publishing House, Beijing, 1994.

(4) Wallin MT, Culpepper WJ, Campbell JD, et al. The prevalence of MS in the United States: a population-based estimate using health claims data. *Neurology* 2019;92:e1029–e1040.

(5) Jason Jishun Hao, Wei Cheng, and Ming Liu et al, Treatment of Multiple Sclerosis with Chinese Scalp Acupuncture

Glob Adv Health Med. 2013 Jan; 2(1): 8–13.

Published online 2013 Jan 1. doi: 10.7453/gahmj.2013.2.1.002

(6, 7) World Health Organization *Atlas: multiple sclerosis resources in the world, 2008.* Geneva, Switzerland: WHO Library Cataloguing in Publication Data; 2008

(8) WebMD.com [Internet] Cerebral palsy – topic overview. Cited 6 Feb 2008. Available from: http://children.webmd.com/tc/cerebral-palsy-topic-overview

(9, 10) United Cerebral Palsy Fact Sheet, Cited 6 Feb 2008.

https://ucp.org/wp-content/uploads/2022/02/cp-fact-sheet.pdf

(11) Beukelman DR, Mirenda P. *Augmentative and alternative communication: management of severe communication disorders in children and adults.* 2nd ed Baltimore: Paul H. Brookes Publishing Co; 1999. p. 246–99

(12) Fact About Cerebral Palsy, cited 28 Feb. 2023 from https://cerebralpalsy.org.au/our-research/about-cerebral-palsy/what-is-cerebral-palsy/facts-about-cerebral-palsy/

(13) CDC's Morbidity and Mortality Weekly Report (January 30, 2004): "Economic Costs Associated with Mental Retardation, Cerebral Palsy, Hearing Loss, and Vision Impairment — United States, 2003"

(14) Jason Jishun Hao and Linda Lingzhi Hao, *Chinese Scalp Acupuncture*, Blue Poppy Press, 2011, p 71-72

(15) Vos T, Allen C, Arora M, Barber RM, Bhutta ZA, Brown A, et al. (GBD 2015 Disease and Injury Incidence and Prevalence Collaborators) (8 October 2016)

(16) "Traumatic brain injury." Centers for Disease Control and Prevention, National Center for Injury Prevention and Control. 2007.

(17) Erlenwein J, Diers M, Ernst J, Schulz F, Petzke F. Clinical updates on phantom limb pain. *Pain Rep.* 2021;6(1):e888. Published 2021 Jan 15.

(18) Centers for Disease Control and COVID, Cited 3 Feb. 2023. Available from: www.cdc.gov/covid/documents/cp.pdf

(19) World Health Organization and Covid, Cited 3 Feb. 2023. Available from: htt;//covid19.who.int/ WHO Coronavirus (COVID-19) Dashboard

(20) C Saunders, A new paradigm is needed to explain long COVID. *Lancet Respir Med.* 2023 Feb;11(2):e12-e13.

(21) Jia, Huai-yu et al., *Scalp Acupuncture Therapy*, People's Medical Publishing House, Beijing, 1994, p. 92-97

(22) Larsen, Stephen, *The Healing Power of Neurofeedback*, Healing Arts Press, Rochester, VT, 2006, p. xiii-xv

(23) Brown, David, "Brain Rebuilding," *Albuquerque Journal*, January 31, 2011, p. C-1

(24) Doidge, Norman, *The Brain That Changes Itself,* Penguin Group, Inc., New York, 2007, p. xix

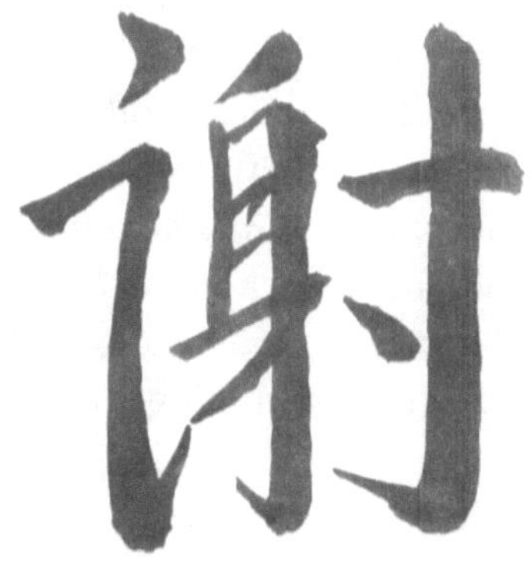

ACKNOWLEDGMENTS

I acknowledge, with sincere thanks, my teachers, colleagues, friends, and family who helped me write my first book in English focusing on patient stories.

I feel so grateful and blessed that I received my professional training directly from Jiao Shunfa, the founder of Chinese scalp acupuncture, and Sun Shentian, the grand master of Chinese medicine, and Yu Zhishun, famous professors of research and development in scalp acupuncture.

I would like to express heartfelt gratitude for the integrity of Karen Bomm, a publishing strategist whom I was referred to. She inspired me to share my unique story, and kept me laser-focused on writing about the effective results I provide for patients through my art and passion for this new, growing technique called neuro-acupuncture.

Jeff Braucher, my editor, helped each story stay true to its voice. He applied the clarity, conciseness, consistency, and word choice needed for both patients and practitioners to enjoy reading this book. Maya Magee Sutton was without a doubt my key assistant in preparing the required early draft before the final edits were applied. Thank you, both.

Diane Rigoli is pleasant and direct in ways that serviced our creative ideas necessary to deliver a quality book design within a pressing timeline. Her graphic touches enhanced every part of my book, guiding the reader eloquently through each uplifting story.

I would like to recognize all the acupuncture practitioners, students, friends, and patients who have encouraged me to persevere in this task. Their positive attitudes and interest gave this book life so it could aid those searching for real solutions to their health challenges.

Finally, this book would not have come into being without my parents, my brothers, my wife, my son, and my daughter in-law. Their continuous encouragement, support, advice, and inspiration gave me the strength to commit to this book project, the first in a series of books I plan to write.

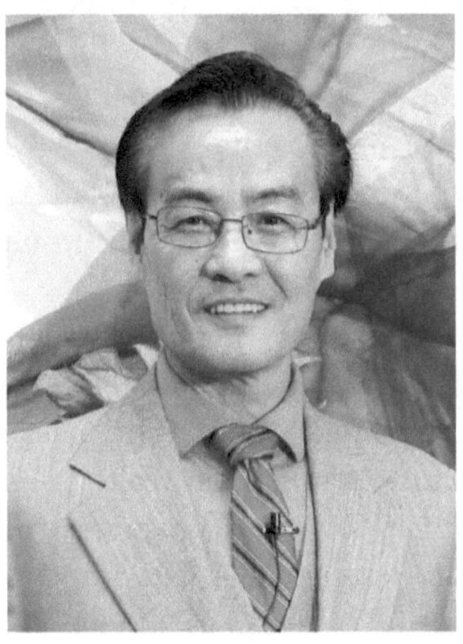

ABOUT THE AUTHOR

Jason Jishun Hao, DOM, is the founder and president of the Neuro-Acupuncture Institute in the USA. For more than 40 years, Dr. Hao has been practicing and researching scalp acupuncture, and since 1989 he has been teaching classes and seminars in the US.

Published in many medical books and journals, Dr. Hao has had articles written about him over past 40 years. He is the co-author of *Chinese Scalp Acupuncture and Professional English for Traditional Chinese Medicine.*

Jason Hao is editor-in-chief and translator-in-chief for the textbook *Acupuncture and Moxibustion,* published by World Federation of Chinese Medicine Societies. He is vice editor-in-chief for the textbook *Stress Response and Syndromes of Traditional Chinese Medicine.* He has also contributed to many integrative medical books, including *Pain Procedures in Clinical Practice,* and *The Scientific Basis of Integrative Health, and Acupuncture for Brain.*

Dr. Hao has voluntarily offered his services to advance the medical profession and inform the public. He currently serves as the vice-chairman for the education guiding committee and vice president of the translating committee of World Federation of Chinese Medicine Societies. He was former chairman of the acupuncture committee at the National Certification Commission of Acupuncture and Oriental Medicine (NCCAOM), former president of New Mexico Chinese School of Arts and Language, and former examiner for the license examination of doctor of oriental medicine in New Mexico.

Jason Hao has taught numerous seminars on neuro-acupuncture in Denmark, the Netherlands, German, Italy, Hungary, Australia, China, and Dubai in the past 40 years. He gave a neuro-acupuncture seminar at Walter Reed Medical Center in Washington, DC, where he successfully demonstrated neuro-acupuncture treatment of CRPS and phantom pain for veterans.

He specializes in treating neurological disorders such as stroke, multiple sclerosis, traumatic brain injury, PTSD, cerebral palsy, autism, complex regional pain, phantom pain, and long COVID-19 disorders. Jason Hao has helped many patients recover from their neurological disorders. For over 33 years, the American media (newspapers, journals, television) has followed him to report his successful cases and stories. Released in May 2022, the documentary film *Return to Life* by Doug Dearth focuses on Jason Hao and his wife, Linda Hao, demonstrating their neuro-acupuncture treatments.

Dr. Hao will travel and teach neuro-acupuncture in many countries throughout Europe in the summer of 2023, including England, France, Italy, and Switzerland. A new documentary film that tells his story is titled *Cowboy Needleman,* which is scheduled to be released in 2023.

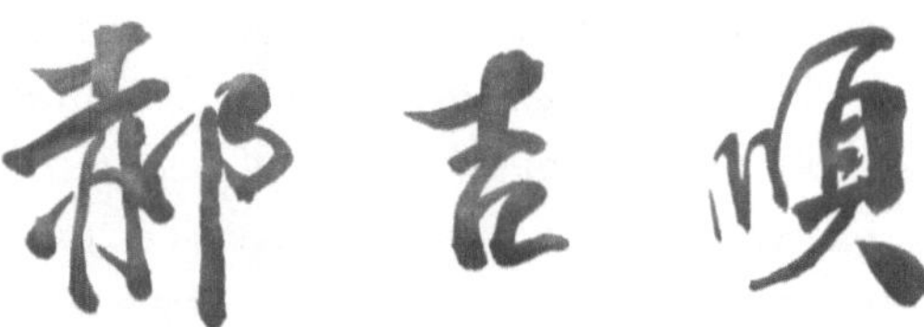

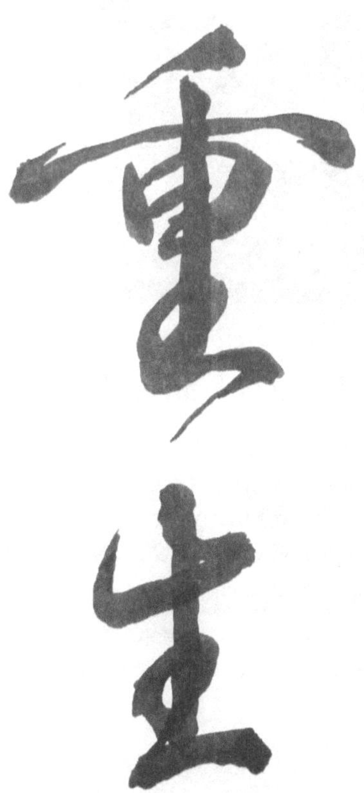

NEURO-ACUPUNCTURE INSTITUTE

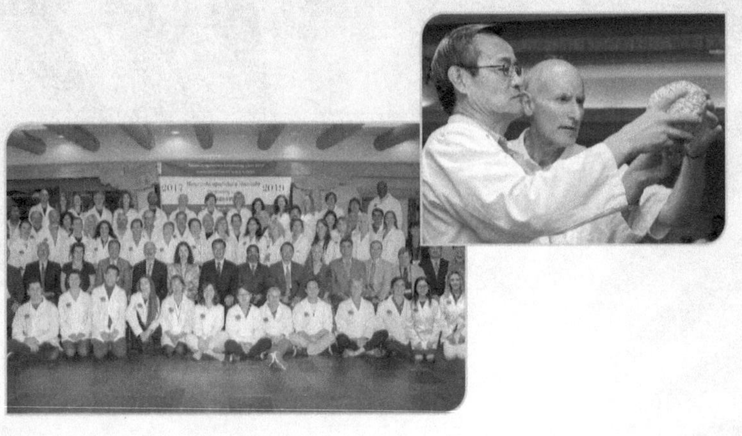

MISSION STATEMENT

THE NEURO-ACUPUNCTURE INSTITUTE, INC. is dedicated to clinical training and treatment of neurological disorders in an integrative medical setting. The Institute offers further purpose by raising public awareness of neuro-acupuncture procedures and processes to promote education, training and research.

The Neuro-Acupuncture Institute is a 501(c)(3) nonprofit organization. Anyone can make donations to the Neuro-Acupuncture Institute which are tax deductible.

A percentage of the proceeds from sales of this book will be contributed to the Neuro-Acupuncture Institute.

Neuro-AcupunctureInstitute.org

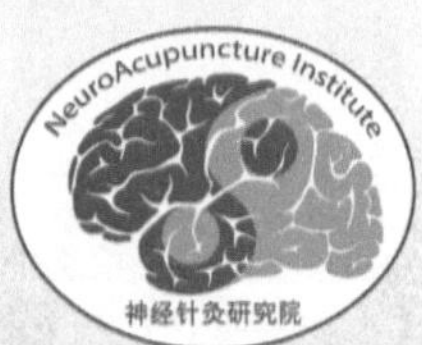

A Neuro-Acupuncture Patient Story Series

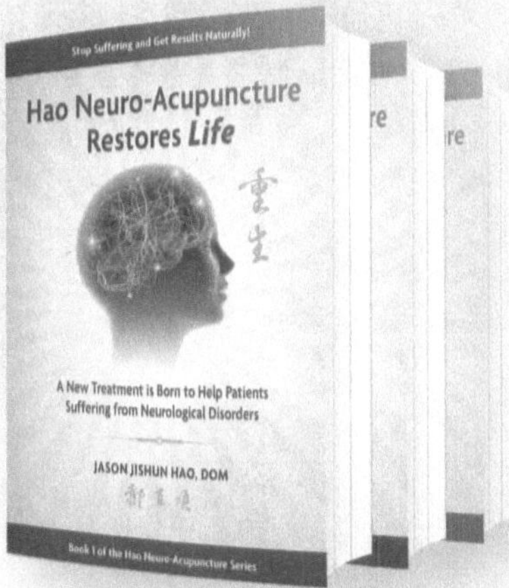

HaoNeuro-AcupuncturePress.com

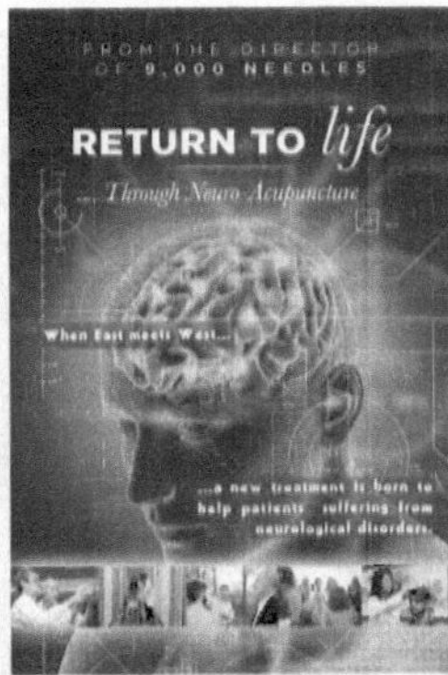

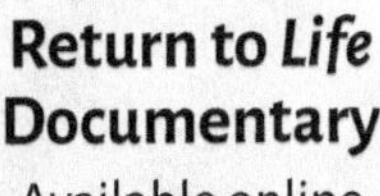

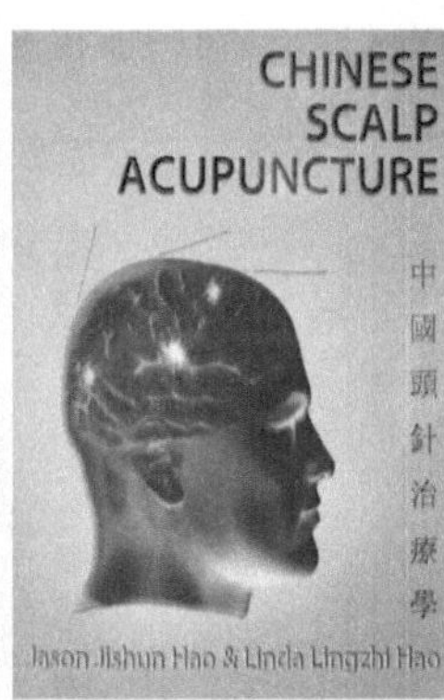

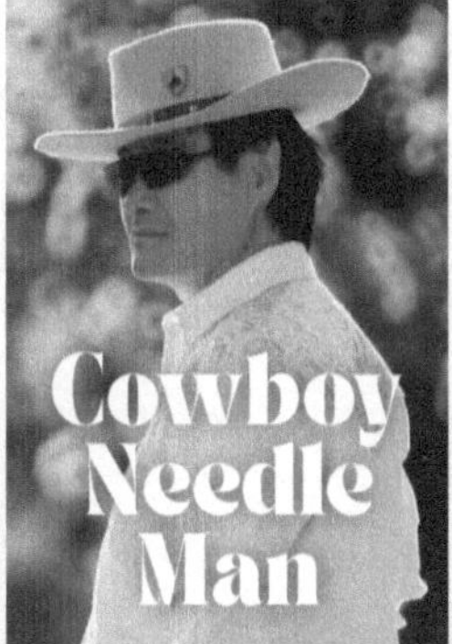

Return to *Life* Documentary

Available online

Chinese Scalp Acupuncture

Training Manual for Doctors and DOM's

New Movie Cowboy Needle Man

Coming soon

www.ingramcontent.com/pod-product-compliance
Lightning Source LLC
Chambersburg PA
CBHW021547150726
47990CB00006B/2431